The
Homeopathic
Conversation

The Art of
Taking the Case

Dr Brian Kaplan MBBCh. FFHom.

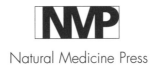

Natural Medicine Press

Where the love of man is,
there also is love of this Art.
(Hippocrates)

The Homeopathic Conversation
The Art of Taking the Case

Published by Natural Medicine Press,
140 Harley Street, London W1G 7LB
www.drkaplan.co.uk
nmp@blueyonder.co.uk

Second edition 2002, Reprinted 2005

British Library Cataloguing in Publication Data
A catalogue record for this book is available from the British Library.

ISBN 1 903952 00 X

Cover design and image by Ergo at www.ergo-id.com

Typeset by Robin Giddings, robinartwork@yahoo.co.uk
Printed and bound by Bell & Bain Ltd., Glasgow

Dedicated to my teachers,
students and patients

Contents

Acknowledgements

The patients who taught me what classical homeopathy was all about.

The students who helped me learn how to teach it.

The Faculty of Homeopathy for welcoming me into the fold and
Jo and Mair for making me feel at home when I arrived in 1982.

My teachers: everyone at the Royal London Homoeopathic Hospital who
taught me – Drs Jenkins, Kennedy, Clover, Davies, English, Lessell and Twentyman –
I learned from you all.

Dr Marianne Harling, a gentlewoman of homoeopathy if ever there was one.

My colleagues at HPTG (David Curtin, David Owen, Alice Greene, Charles Forsyth,
John Saxton and Peter Gregory) and Mary and Hilary of course.

Dr Eric Ledermann, who taught me by word and example,
the true measure of a doctor – authenticity.

George Vithoulkas for those wonderful seminars and meetings in Alonissos.

Dr Andrew Lockie, who always encouraged me to write.

Tony Pinkus, for good advice and some great talks in your car
as well as all those fabulous homeopathic dinners.

Dr Dapinder Rattan Singh for seemingly unlimited generosity of spirit,
not to mention those great meals!

Dr Roger Neighbour for writing one of the best books ever on General Practice
and being so helpful and friendly on the phone.

John and Nick Churchill for reading the manuscript
and for always being available for advice.

Dana Ullman, for giving me a lot of extremely useful feedback
on the manuscript and general encouragement for the project.

Dr Claire Pickin for the wonderful story.

Jeremy Sherr for allowing me to quote his wise words on case-taking.

Frances Treuherz for always being so helpful and cheerful on the phone.

Colin, David, John, Maura, Sue and everyone else 'on the street'.
Special thanks to you, Colin, for the kind words and encouragement.

Mr Mark Ornstein for being the friendliest surgeon around
and Harris Sidelsky for being so generous.

Professor Alan Widgerow, Mr Dev Basra and Dar for being there when it mattered.

Arnold Brown for the friendship, the laughter, the irony and especially that joke...

Frank Farrelly for the laughs, the love and first pointing out how homeopathic Provocative Therapy really is.

Dr Hans Zwemke, (one of the world's most under-rated classical homeopaths) for being a true friend, and honouring me by inviting me to teach on this subject in Berlin – and for approving of the manuscript, which meant a lot to me.

Man Xing, for that e-mail about the manuscript.
It meant more to me than you may think.

Robin Shohet, for advising me to write in 'conversational style' I got some flak for it, but I still think you were right. Thanks too for all the wonderful supervison.

Richard Joseph, for choosing this book for the 'new way' and for always being so warm and friendly, and Jane Elliot and the team for living with me in the 'pressure cooker'.

Russell Caplan, of MaCaplan Computer Consultancy for being such a good friend to me and doctor (always on call) to my computer.

Enid Segal, for being a friend and librarian at the BHA on a day when the heat was really on.

Fred and the boychiks at the shtiebl.

Ruth, Adrianna (Zsa-Zsa), and Anna Paula for looking after Jonah, when his parents were obsessed with the book.

Bill and Julie Petrie for useful feedback and being good friends.

Tessa Bilder for insightful feedback and Jem for finding that definition!

Jennifer and Carlos for the spirit and body work.

Anthony Kingsley for useful feedback and being a good friend and neighbour.

Marc Suttner, great friend and aspirant geek, but always 'the dude'.

Mike Mandelbaum, friend and confederate, for support throughout and for igniting the second phase of the project.

My parents-in-law, Anton and June for general support with the project and letting me write and holiday in your wonderful flat.

My late colleague and friend, Lee Holland.
I thought a lot about our chats while writing this....

My sisters Cathy and Meg for supporting the project in many different ways.

My late father, David, who left me with the gift of enthusiasm for life.
Who can ask for more than that?

My mother, Rick and her husband, Nat, for the happy working holidays at your home. Thanks for feeding me as I worked and the happy spirit in the house.
It really kept me going ...

My son, Jonah, for putting up with me when in 'mad author mode' and those hugs.

Hephzibah, my lovely wife, for showing me the role of images and art therapy in homeopathy as well as many expert contributions – but more for being who you are and being there for me.

Preface

It took me nearly two decades to realise something obvious about classical homeopathy – the conversations we have with our patients are the most important part of the whole process.

Why is this so obvious? Picture in your mind a homeopath who has an encyclopaedic knowledge of the materia medica, an intelligent and flexible approach to case analysis, including the use of computers and a comprehensive, homeopathic library. However, this homeopath is simply not very good company. Patients feel slightly uneasy in his consulting room and his friends and family have always found it a little hard 'getting through' to him.

Now picture in your mind another homeopath. This one is the sort of person everyone just can't help opening up to. He is just so understanding and sympathetic. Such a good listener. His only problem is that he doesn't know much about homeopathy. He knows what sort of information you need to get from your consultations but as for the materia medica, well, there are just so many remedies, how on earth can anybody expect him to remember any of them. As for books on homeopathic theory, they are just so hard to read.

If you had to make a choice, which of these two would you consult? It has to be the latter for one good reason. The homeopath who is able to take good case histories at least has a chance of finding your remedy. He is able to leave the consulting room with your main symptoms, in particular your emotional profile. He can use repertories, computers and the materia medica to help him find a remedy to match what he knows about you. He can phone up a colleague, better versed in the materia medica, and ask for advice or take your case to a supervision group.

As for the former homeopath, I guess he will be left wondering why he doesn't have much of a practice considering the thousands of hours he has spent studying homeopathy. And why do his remedies just not seem to work? He knows their drug pictures so well. Why can't he find any patients to fit them?

The sad truth is that such a 'homeopath' might as well give up homeopathy and go and study surgery or massage. Maybe his talent always was in his hands.

People become homeopaths for different reasons. Some are so grateful for what a remedy did for them that they become determined to study this amazing subject. Others are fascinated by homeopathic theory. There are those who are smitten by the idea that every mineral, metal, plant, poison or animal secretion has specific healing qualities that can potentially be matched to the whole of the patient physically and psychologically. There are even those, like Hering, who studied homeopathy in order to refute it but ended up falling in love with it. Few students of homeopathy choose the discipline because they are good listeners and enjoy talking to patients.

The ability to listen well and say the right thing at the right moment is central to the homeopathic process. It is surprising that so little has been written about taking the case and the homeopath-patient relationship.

This book is an attempt to draw attention to what actually happens in the homeopathic clinic. To do this it is necessary to examine what is going on in the mind of the patient, the mind of the homeopath and in the space between them. Although homeopaths have not, until quite recently, focused on the practitioner-patient relationship, the disciplines of psychotherapy and counselling have always recognised that relationship to be a vital factor in the prognosis of the patient. It is the contention of this book that this relationship is even more vital in homeopathy, not only because we have less time to spend with our patients than counsellors and psychotherapists do, but because the reward for effective communication between homeopath and patient is the prescription of the correct remedy.

The value of the correct prescription is inestimable and yet it is not the only reason for learning to have more authentic conversations with patients. The syndrome of 'burnout' is far from uncommon among homeopaths. Many of us end up feeling drained by our patients. It can be a heavy burden being a homeopath. We know the potential of our remedies but we have to live with the shadow of feeling guilty about patients suffering because we have not been able to find the right remedy. As we learn to have more meaningful conversations with our patients, this guilt gradually diminishes and the responsibility for finding the remedy begins to be shared by homeopath and patient.

I have written this book for fellow homeopaths and homeopathic students alike. We are all students of homeopathy and I have yet to meet anyone who claims to have mastered the materia medica or the taking of the case. It takes decades of both study and clinical practice to make serious inroads into the materia medica and there are no short cuts. The study of books on homeopathic theory, especially the *Organon*, can be inspiring, but are only fully appreciated after many years of consulting.

Fortunately, when it comes to taking the case, I feel that it is possible to make some progress quite quickly if the teachers and students of homeopathy choose to focus on this aspect of homeopathy from the very beginning of any course of training. If anything, it can be a lot more fun than trying to memorise the materia medica. Taking the case should be of equal interest to us all. Experience in the clinic is the greatest teacher, but when it comes to communicating with patients, it is quite possible for the 'master' to learn something from the 'absolute beginner'. This is because authentic conversation is more about life itself than it is about the homeopathic consultation.

This book is the result of a long, personal journey of exploration into anything that I felt could help me communicate better with patients. This journey included forays into psychotherapy and psychoanalytic theory, counselling, philosophy, and, of course, what both homeopaths and orthodox doctors had to say about the practitioner-patient relationship. I have tried to collate here only what I consider to be of direct relevance to the homeopathic paradigm. This is not to say that the rest of the journey was a waste of time. I found psychoanalytic theory, for example, fascinating, perplexing and elitist – but finally, amusing.

I have deliberately been transparent about my own learning process in the hope that others will choose to do the same. I have attended so many homeopathic seminars and masterclasses where I have been dying to ask the teacher about what happens in the consulting room. It has nearly always seemed inappropriate to do so as the subject matter of these courses always seems to be about theory, case analysis and the materia medica. This needs to change as case-taking skills are at least as important as these aspects of homeopathy.

As we live in politically correct times, I guess I should give the usual explanation for the use of the masculine form of the third person pronoun for the homeopath. When describing hypothetical consultations I thought long and hard about the alternatives but decided 's/he' looked clumsy and contrived, 'she' patronising and an alternation of 'he' and 'she' a mess.

As for the spelling of 'homeopath', publishing conventions and usage in databases and search engines dictate that I use this modern form, despite my preference for the more traditional version, 'homoeopath'. However, this latter is retained if it is part of a proper name for an institution or if it appears in the title of a book.

Finally I would like to say something about the style in which this book is written. If it feels chatty and a little irreverent at times, please know that this is quite deliberate. I wanted the book to feel a bit like a conversation between reader and writer. I apologise that this conversation had to take the form of a monologue but what could I do? Still, the world of homeopathy is quite small and perhaps one day we may meet face to face and enjoy a real homeopathic conversation.

Chapter 1

Becoming a Doctor

Do you want to help sick people? Be a doctor, healer or carer? Do you want to be a good homeopath? You do? Why?

Why of all the jobs on earth would you choose one that invites into your living space people who are in discomfort, pain, mental anguish or may even be dying?

It certainly isn't the easiest way to make a living and specialising in homeopathy doesn't make it any easier. As a homeopath, you allow people to come into your life and unload in great detail the most painful parts of their lives right on to you and into the space you have provided for them. This book is about you, your patients and what happens between you. As you have been yourself for longer than you have been interested in homeopathy it would seem logical to start with yourself. So why do you want to be a good homeopath?

Okay then, I will answer the question myself and try to show you why this process of understanding is necessary.

At the age of 15 I decided that I wanted to be a doctor. I was more or less at the top of my class at school and confident or arrogant enough to think I could choose any profession that I fancied. I remember very well the thought processes that accompanied this momentous decision. 'If I become a doctor, I will be able to help people. So wherever I am in the world I can be useful. I will be needed. Even if I change as a person, surely those simple facts will remain. So I will study hard at school in order to get into medical school.' And that is exactly what happened. But of course I had omitted to ask the most important question of all. Why did I want to be needed? Especially at that age. Looking back now I can understand a lot more. For one thing I was lonely. My school, an awful, boys-only affair that all but derided academic achievement in favour of what really counted (rugby and cricket) was not a happy place for me. No girlfriend, no girls in the school. Yes, of course I had a need to be needed. But was this a good basis to make one of the most important decisions of my life? At the time it didn't even occur to me. I had decided to become a doctor and that was that. It would be at least two decades before I took a good look at the child that made the decision that sent my life spiralling into medical school and later on into homeopathy.

The programme at my medical school was six years long. First year was on a beautiful campus with all the other students, the ones studying subjects like drama, psychology, languages, politics and so on. The first year in our course was devoted to the basic sciences: physics, chemistry, biology, as well as a bit of maths and sociology. It was fun to be there and the subjects we were reading, especially physics, had that simple purity and beauty that are peculiar to the first year of the study of a basic science. My grades were good and I thoroughly enjoyed campus life. I looked forward to the next stage of the long adventure. A horrible shock was waiting for me.

Second-year medicine meant removal from that beautiful green-lawned campus to an ugly building near the teaching hospital. First year had been a simple platform (dispensed with at most European medical schools) for the real business of becoming a doctor. Don't be misled by the fact that this place was near the hospital. It would be another two years before I would even see a patient. But I was on my way to becoming a doctor. What I did not know was that the process my medical school used to achieve this was not that different from breaking in a horse. My desire to become a helper or carer or doctor was about to receive its sternest challenge. On the first day of second-year medical school I was introduced to the only teacher I would see six days a week for a whole year, a dead man lying supine on a dissecting table. At medical school we called such people cadavers.

One of my most enduring memories of medical school was the ceremony held to mark the start of our work in the dissecting halls. Desmond Tutu, then an Anglican bishop, was invited to make a short address to us. He expressed himself simply and asked us humbly to offer thanks to the 50 or so dead people covered in sheets that lay on tables in front of us. Some may have donated their bodies to science but I fear that in the South Africa of the 1970s most would have been unclaimed bodies. We had been allocated one cadaver per four students and would spend the greater part of six days a week dissecting it.

The purpose of dissecting a cadaver is to study anatomy. There is no doubt whatsoever that this is the best way to become an anatomist. Whether several hours a day of immersing oneself in a dead body is the best way to start training a doctor is a moot point. Perhaps it is also important to talk to some live patients and ask them about how they experienced being ill. It would have been no problem to find volunteers for this. It would have been therapeutic for the patients themselves to talk to a sympathetic ear even if it wasn't attached to the head of a person with a degree in medicine. To be fair, some medical schools are starting to realise this now and encouraging medical students at an early stage of their education to talk to patients in wards.

There are those that think that a boy or girl who cuts up a frog or bird is a prospective physician. In first-year biology, I had thrown away the only dead rat ever given to me. I simply failed to see its role in teaching me to become a doctor. And the smell! But now there was no escape. I would have to participate in cutting up every part, and I mean every part, of this dead man that would stare up at me each day. Or at least while he was still recognisable as a man. I think of him every now and then and with some gratitude. He taught me a lot. It was not his fault that my medical school had an anatomy programme that brutalised its students both in its demands and in the testing of our knowledge of absurd detail. For surgeons this is necessary but for almost every other area of medicine it was both unnecessary and cruel. And if you couldn't take the pressure, well there were always other things to do with your life. Not every horse can become a racehorse.

I saw a few lovely people who could have become good family doctors or psychiatrists or homeopaths drop out, or be thrown out after failing too badly or, even worse, repeat this terrible year. I passed but not without personal cost. The very ideal that had led me to medical school, the desire to help, had receded and been surpassed by the simple desire to survive. Self-preservation – at any cost. And at the end of this challenging year, in which we also studied physiology in the same generally useless but very punishing detail, there would be two more similar years studying subjects like pathology, microbiology and pharmacology to go before I would meet a patient. Six years is a long time when you are 18 years old.

Before I leave second-year medical school there is someone I must mention as he was the only person in all six years at medical school who – besides our cadaver – I really regarded as a teacher. His name is Professor Philip Tobias, a superb anatomist and world-famous anthropologist. As author of the dissection manual, he was more or less responsible for the detailed anatomy we were supposed to remember. However, there was something more to this man than simply being a brilliant anatomist and ground-breaking anthropologist. It was the way he viewed life and the world. His lectures were never less than inspiring simply by way of the context in which he presented the material. I will never forget his lecture to us at the end of the six-year programme. He spoke about how important it was for doctors to be able to smile. Those patients who were not smiling themselves may just be the ones who could most benefit from a smile from the doctor. I remember that remark bringing tears to my eyes. (They are there again as I write this.) Interaction between human beings had been mentioned!

Third year was no improvement; the subjects studied were pathology, microbiology and forensic pathology. We did see patients but only those who had died recently and usually only the parts of them that had been incriminated in their demise. This is how you study gross pathology. Fresh parts of a dead human being are dissected on the slab in front of you so you can see the disease. Interesting for some. And perhaps necessary in moderation for all, but something less than inspiring for a young man who wanted to become a doctor so he could help people. Only another three years to go after this one!

In fourth year we were introduced to the wards and taught to take a medical history and examine patients. This teaching was invaluable and I am very grateful to have had the opportunity to receive it. To be able to interview and examine a patient properly is a skill that is a privilege to acquire. Still, I have some reservations about the way it was taught. The techniques of examination were taught faultlessly. The problem was that nobody mentioned that it might be polite to ask the patient's permission before you put your hands on his body (and this is even more obvious when it is her body). No, the general emphasis was on acquiring useful information in order to arrive at a diagnosis. Investigations may be ordered to assist this and the whole process may essentially be described as mechanistic. Although we were told not to speak about the diastolic heart murmur in bed nine but refer to her as Mrs Robinson, the general talk was very much about murmurs and bruits, enlarged livers and spleens, interesting lumps and bumps, unusual rashes and so on. We were taught medicine much as a mechanic must be taught about motor cars. First, study normal structure and function and then learn how to diagnose any sort of malfunction. Yes, of course it's a lot harder to become a doctor than a mechanic but that may be because the human body is much more complex than a car. Since we don't manufacture human beings, we don't have a definitive work manual. A problem.

Nevertheless I learned something of immense value that year. I was taught that although clinical examination was important and investigations such as blood tests and X-rays are very useful, 75 per cent of diagnoses should be made from the history alone. In other words, talking to your patient was the most important part of clinical medicine. This is even truer for the homeopath but 'homeopathy' was a dirty word for me in those days.

We were taught what questions to ask but not how to ask them. A pity, because how to ask questions, when to ask them and especially when not to ask questions is the very essence of what we can call the art of medicine.

Medical science is a science indeed. A noble science. But science is not enough to make a doctor. Medicine is also an art, an art that takes many decades of experience to learn well. Medical school taught me much too much of the science and little, if anything, of the art of medicine. Considering I was in their clutches for a full six years I feel I am justified in expressing this regret. Five of the six years I was there were especially painful for me because I really needed to start learning the art of medicine, how to talk to patients, take an interest in their lives and start learning what the word 'rapport' means. No, it was just facts, long lists of facts, many of them irrelevant to a general practitioner. It took long, boring hours to memorise these lists and for a young man who wanted to be a doctor because he yearned to 'help people' this was a severe challenge. Why was I so unhappy, even bored? I was becoming a doctor, my life's ambition. Why? It would be many years before I could really answer this important question. Finally, I realised that I was not even being given a taste of what it was like to be a doctor, helper or carer. Had there been one afternoon a week devoted to communication skills, group work, encouragement to express feelings, things might have been different. Nevertheless I stuck it out, hoping that somewhere over the rainbow there would be a place for me as a doctor.

In the final three years we saw patients in the wards but the emphasis was on making a mechanistic diagnosis and applying the standard treatment for patients with that diagnosis. This, I feel now, is the science rather than the art of medicine. Bemused and even a little frightened, I observed some of the doctors who had reached the pinnacle of medical science. Consultants who were in overall charge of whole wards of patients. Academics whose main responsibility was to teach medical students. Most were masters of the science of medicine and this seemed to be the main criterion for acquiring status and authority in the medical world. Now and then someone would pay lip service to how you might talk to a patient, but the emphasis was clearly on making a scientific diagnosis. Some of these medical authorities were naturally humane and this was reflected in the way they spoke to patients and colleagues. Others, I now see quite clearly, although being good clinicians, were suffering from various personality disorders. This, in itself, is not uncommon among doctors and the concept of the 'wounded healer' is now quite well established. The horror of the situation was that a doctor clearly suffering from a personality disorder and either unaware of it or doing nothing about it could quite easily rise to the top of the tree in medicine. Human qualities were simply not the point. Medicine, ladies and gentlemen, is a science.

No wonder I was not enjoying myself. On one occasion, when I was on the paediatric ward, the social science department of the university made us go on video while talking to a volunteer, the mother of a very sick child. Seeing myself on video was a revelation, a huge shock and a fantastic lesson. As the poet Robert Burns wrote:

> O, wad some power the giftie gie us
> To see oursels as ithers see us!
> It wad frae monie a blunder free us,
> An' foolish notion [1]

Alas, this only happened at the end of six years' training and I never got another chance to see myself on video at medical school. It could and probably should have happened in my first few months there and carried on for the full six years. Had this been the case, I might even have enjoyed medical school. I would have understood that I was being taught both the science and the art of medicine and the inspiration of the process of learning the art would have taken much of the pain out of the necessary process of memorising lists of scientific facts.

In this final year I studied very hard. My aim was to do my best to get the most I could of what was on offer and moreover to make sure that I graduated.

Professor Tobias gave his inspiring lecture about the demeanour of a doctor and the importance of smiling. The nightmare of final examinations finally ended. I had passed. I was a doctor! But had I learned anything about helping people? Did I have one per cent of the counselling skills of the average person who answers a helpline on the telephone? Did I know anything at all about psychotherapy, homeopathy or holistic medicine? Had I thought about what the expression 'Physician heal thyself' actually means?

After six arduous years of study the time had come to be a doctor. This was the famous internship or housemanship year about which much has been written in books such as *The House of God* [2] by Samuel Shem. The 110-hour weeks; the 48-hour shifts; bullying, senior doctors and detached consultants. Yes, it is all true, as any doctor will confirm.

Still I am glad to be able to say that I turned out to be a much better doctor than medical student. It was hard, the hours were long, and the taskmasters could be tough. At times I felt that I was being tested again. I remember more than anything what it felt like to be deprived of sleep for very long periods. I would go about my duties like an emotionally wrecked zombie. Anything could make me laugh but just as easily bring tears to my eyes. Would you like a doctor in such a state to treat your seriously ill child?

There were good times too. I was responsible for my own patients (with supervision) and on the whole I handled the year well. I watched as lives were saved by drugs and surgery and was exposed to the full power of mechanistic medicine in treating serious diseases. I could not help being impressed as I saw diseases such as meningitis and pneumonia respond well to biological warfare. I saw smashed bones bolted together, allowing their owners to walk rather than limp for the rest of their lives. I saw sophisticated diagnoses made by great physicians. In 1981 medical science was at the peak of its power (alternative medicine was virtually unheard of) and many previously untreatable conditions (including some cancers) were now being treated without much trouble. On the other hand, I did not enjoy working in a hospital and while I could admire much of what I saw done, I could not see a place for myself anywhere in this whole structure. I felt drawn to nothing except a few weeks' rest. It was December and we would all finish our internships at the end of the month. I was in the cancer ward. Patients were dying every day. My colleagues were all arranging their next jobs, starting, of course, on the first of January. I made no such plans. In fact I came back to the cancer ward on New Year's Day to introduce the poor new interns to the ward. It took the whole morning but then I finally felt free to leave. It was a glorious summer's day and I decided to go for a walk around a lake. I had no job and at that very moment was slipping behind in the medical rat race as the clock ticked. I had no plans for the future and virtually no money. Everything around me looked beautiful, the trees, the lake and all the people I made eye contact with. Far from feeling uncertain about the future I felt strangely optimistic. Even happy.

So I took some time off. It took two-and-a-half weeks before I thought I should be working again. Doing nothing was making me feel guilty at some level, particularly because all my peers were now starting new jobs in their chosen specialities. I had no particular ambition and no enthusiasm for any branch of medicine I had encountered so far. I liked obstetrics. Watching my first birth had been a momentous occasion and I was also fortunate that a friend had forced me to read Frederik Leboyer's masterpiece, *Birth Without Violence,*[3] at that time. It made a profound impression on me. His compassion and respect for the neonate's first few minutes on earth seemed so clear and so obvious and so contrary to what I saw practised at the time. But gynaecology and obstetrics were not for me. For one thing I am not a natural-born surgeon. More to the point, I realised that it was midwives rather than doctors that really get involved in the miracle of birth. The art of obstetrics is how and when not to get involved, but there are wonderful books by Leboyer, Odent and others on the elegance of natural childbirth. An obstetrician helps the difficult deliveries, performs Caesarean sections and of course all the gynaecological operations. So there was no real home for me there either. Psychiatry had always interested me but there was no specialisation in psychotherapy available for doctors, and five more years of conventional mechanistic medicine felt unappealing. I also found it amazing that a specialisation in psychiatry did not even include psychotherapy skills. There was certainly no obligation to be in psychotherapy yourself. I had even heard a rumour that it was actually slightly frowned upon! No place for me there either.

I had always been interested in yoga, particularly hatha yoga which deals with the physical postures known as asanas. They seemed more sophisticated than conventional aerobic and calisthenic exercises and I felt very well after attending some classes. One day I wandered into a New Age-type bookshop in the middle of Johannesburg and browsed. There was a sale on and a book caught my eye. It was entitled *Homoeopathy: An Introductory Guide* by a Dr Gordon-Ross,[4] but that is not what had drawn my attention.

I'd seen the letters MBBS after the author's name. That was my qualification. Bachelor of medicine, bachelor of surgery. A doctor! A doctor practising homeopathic medicine? It was a huge shock and I am ashamed to say that I almost tossed the book back in contempt. But it was really cheap; they were giving it away. I bought it and read it. The book is written in a semi-autobiographical style and it was the personal stuff that really got to me. Of course the author wrote a little about the theory and practice of homeopathy and about some of the medicines but this is not what drew my attention. What captivated me was that it was obvious, almost from the first page, that this doctor had enjoyed his life as a homeopathic doctor. He enthused about the power of homeopathic remedies and how they had helped him become a more effective and happier general practitioner. At the time I was amazed and inspired by everything in the book. The fascinating history of homeopathy, the theory and practice and the preparation and power of the remedies themselves.

As I read the short paperback book, I experienced something quite wonderful. The idealism that had made me decide to be a doctor started to rouse itself. I felt the old enthusiasm about being a carer or helper as a distinct physical sensation. I realise now that it had little to do with the homeopathic theory and medicines and everything to do with the quality of relationship that could exist between homeopath and patient. At the age of 16 I had naively hoped for something like what was described in this book. I had seen nothing like it at medical school. Of course I had been taught the importance of taking a good history. I had even been told that most medical diagnoses could probably be made from the history alone. However, a medical history has the aim of beginning the process of diagnosing disease. Most of what the patient says is considered of little importance in this regard. The doctor is waiting for vital clues that are symptoms of a specific disease. He may express some interest in other information about the patient's life but it is of far less importance. The fact that a patient with asthma may have a specific phobia about high places or travelling in aeroplanes may be of some interest but will not make a difference to the diagnosis or the treatment. Although the orthodox textbooks recommend that we let the patient tell his or her story in their own words, in practice many direct questions are asked in a standard medical history in order to establish whether or not a patient has a specific symptom. For example, a doctor might directly ask a patient whether he ever wakes up at night needing to go to the window to breathe fresh air. This is known as paroxysmal nocturnal dyspnoea and is a symptom of heart failure. Of course in psychiatry things were a little different but diagnosis of a disease was still the most important objective. Correct diagnosis leads to appropriate medication.

I had always enjoyed talking to patients about their lives in general, their families and their jobs, forgetting for a few moments the world of medical diagnoses. And now a medical doctor was telling me that this general information about the patient's physical and mental state was the very essence of homeopathic medicine! You needed to know as much as possible about your patient's life. Careful listening was required. Anything the patient said could be of the utmost importance in choosing the right remedy. The passion with which a patient said something was to be taken very seriously and weighted accordingly when choosing a medicine. I had always known that bedside manner was important and that patients preferred to be treated as human beings rather than organic mechanisms. But what I read here was somewhat different. The better I understood my patient as a person, the better my chances were of helping him with homeopathy, both physically and psychologically. This was a huge revelation to me. And if this actually worked? Then it would be necessary for me to have quite a different type of conversation with my patient. A homeopathic conversation. Slowly I began to realise that I was compelled to investigate further. If homeopathy worked, and this was a big 'if' as I had heard it disparaged many times, then it was the closest vocation ever described to my original idea of what it was to be a doctor.

At the end of the book the author suggested that any young doctor wanting to learn more about homeopathy should write to the Faculty of Homoeopathy in London, England, for more information. Nothing could stop me writing immediately, and somehow I sensed that life would never be the same again.

Half of me was simply curious, the other half excited because it sensed that an adventure was about to start. I received a letter fairly promptly offering me the chance to apply for a six-month full-time course at the Royal London Homoeopathic Hospital. I wrote back saying I was interested and would come over and find out more.

A few months later I was in England. It was the first time I had ever left Africa. It was the summer of 1982 and Queen's Square was blooming. I looked up at the building called the Royal London Homoeopathic Hospital. What on earth was I doing?

Chapter 2

Discovering Homeopathy

According to the testimony of all ages, no occupation is more unanimously declared to be a conjectural art than medicine; consequently none has less right to refuse a searching enquiry as to whether it is well founded than it, on which man's health, his most precious possession on earth, depends.

(Hahnemann: opening paragraph of the preface
to the first edition of the Organon, 1810)[5]

On looking back at my introduction to homeopathy, I realise how fortunate I was in many respects. We were eight doctors all beginning a new chapter in our lives, all of us hoping to find something in homeopathy that we knew we needed but had not been able to find in our medical lives. Mavericks perhaps, but I felt more at home in that class than I had ever felt in all my years of nursery school, school, and medical school.

I loved our tutorial room. It was the library of the Faculty of Homoeopathy which was right next door to the Royal London Homoeopathic Hospital. I could not have wished for a better place to learn homeopathy. It was a small room with a beautiful big table around which the eight of us sat for tutorials or general study. The walls of this room were covered with exquisite wooden bookcases bursting with homeopathic books and journals dating back well into the 19th century. Many of these books were rare or out of print. Although I did not appreciate it fully at the time, this was a remarkable and unique environment in which to study homeopathy. I could lean back in my chair, look up a remedy in Hahnemann's *Materia Medica Pura*[6] or Hering's *Guiding Symptoms*[7] or Allen or Hughes or so many others. The collection comprised nearly all the homeopathic literature ever written. We and our tutors not only had access on a daily basis to one of the best homeopathic libraries in the world but we met in that very library every day. This was indeed a privilege and a joy.

There was no particular 'method' of homeopathy advocated by the Faculty. Different teachers had different ideas on how to practise homeopathy and in a way that was fine with me. It was time for me to start thinking for myself rather than being given lists to memorise. I was given an excellent introduction to the history of homeopathy, together with some teaching on the *Organon*, materia medicae, and how to repertorise. Although some lecturers were classical homeopaths, others were influenced by anthroposophy and other schools of thought. It was more or less up to the student to decide who to be influenced by. It was exhilarating simply to study on my own terms. This at last felt like a university rather than a technical college. It was a special time in my life and I could write a lot more about it; however, that is not the point of this book but I remain immensely grateful to all my teachers. While I learned a lot of homeopathic theory and materia medica in those six months, I learned practically nothing about how to take the homeopathic case. Of course I was advised not to put words in the patient's mouth and that unsolicited information was much more valuable than answers to direct questions. I was certainly taught the basics very well. I learned what information from the patient was most useful, how to translate this into homeopathic language and how to use repertories and the materia medica to find a remedy that suited the patient. In other words I learned exactly what information I needed from my patient to be able to make an effective prescription. Unfortunately I was not taught anything of the art of eliciting this information from a patient.

I cannot blame anyone for this because none of the books lining the walls around me had much to say about this subject either. Only one piece of advice was consistently emphasised and that was to let the patient tell you his story in his own words. Don't say much yourself other than non-committal lines like 'Anything else?'. Useful general advice but, as I subsequently discovered, there is a lot more to the art of taking the homeopathic history than that.

I immersed myself totally in homeopathy for six months and studied the materia medica and homeopathic theory very hard indeed for the whole time. I passed the exam for membership of the Faculty of Homoeopathy, one of the very few recognised qualifications in homeopathy for doctors. Now I really was ready to start treating patients. Or so I thought!

Beginner's luck is well known in homeopathy. It's almost as if homeopathy gives its young student a few good results to keep him interested and enthusiastic. I once heard a homeopathic anecdote that went something like this: 'Initially you get a few encouraging results and then you enter a vast desert with no oasis in sight, from which it takes many years to emerge.'

As a colleague once ruefully admitted: 'It only takes three patients in a row telling you there has been no improvement to make you question what you are doing.'

So I attended short homeopathic seminars all over the world to try and learn more. And I learned more of the same. More case analysis and more detailed materia medica. I met George Vithoulkas and was enormously influenced by his encyclopaedic knowledge of materia medica and logical approach to case analysis. I was also impressed and moved by the way he took the case. When talking to patients, his state of consciousness seemed to change. There was an acceptance of the patient's whole being and total focus on what he was saying, doing and being, in the moment. It seemed to me that during consultations, much of who he was as a person disappeared, leaving only the receiver, the listener and the homeopath.

At his school of homeopathy in Alonissos, Greece, I came into contact with many young and enthusiastic classical homeopaths, many of whom are well-known teachers of the present time. It was exhilarating to be in such company and my prescribing definitely improved. I kept showing up at these conferences for many years.

I also tried to sit in with many homeopaths and watch the different styles of taking the case, analysing and prescribing. I watched some very skilled history takers and also some very mechanical interrogations.

I learned a great deal from Dr Eric Ledermann, who I had met during my time at the homeopathic hospital. He is not a classical homeopath but knew a great deal of materia medica. Some might call him a 'keynote prescriber'. Much more importantly he was practising as a psychiatrist and gifted psychotherapist. I attended his clinic every Thursday for at least a year and attended his group psychotherapy sessions as a member/observer every Tuesday night. He would ask me questions like 'What did you think of what I said to that patient when…?' And I was not allowed to get away with non-committal answers. I read his books on his own method of existential psychotherapy and medical philosophy and had the chance to question him every week about his ideas. We also discussed psychological pioneers such as Freud, Jung and Adler, as well as philosophers such as Kant, Husserl, Jaspers and Buber among many. This was a wonderful education because it stimulated me to think about what I thought I was doing as a homeopath and a doctor. It embodied much that had been missing from my education at medical school.

Dr Ledermann prescribed homeopathic remedies at every clinic, sometimes with great success, but psychiatry and especially medical philosophy and ethics were his great passions. They became important to me too and my discussions with him were the sort of education I had always hankered after. Learning had finally become a pleasure.

So at this stage I could only count three really inspirational teachers in my whole education as a doctor. Philip Tobias at medical school for sheer inspiration as a great teacher and intellectual giant; George Vithoulkas for his enthusiasm and beautifully logical approach to classical homeopathy; and Eric Ledermann for dragging me into the world of medical philosophy, ethics and psychotherapy. I had learned from nearly all my teachers but the time spent with these three were important landmarks in my life.

After attending many seminars by famous teachers over many years, an important fact slowly began to dawn on me. I could learn more and more about homeopathic remedies and analysing the case all my life but what was I analysing? If I had not obtained the essential information from my patient I could study the case for weeks and consult all the homeopathic books in the library and ask advice from my most esteemed colleagues, but I would have little chance of finding the correct remedy.

On the other hand if I was able to elicit the most important information from my patient and hardly knew *any* materia medica and homeopathic theory I would have a reasonable chance of finding the right homeopathic remedy. I could consult books, use computer programmes and ask the advice of colleagues. In other words if I had taken a bad case history, no amount of homeopathic knowledge could help me. However, if I had taken the case well, I still had a reasonable chance of success. So why was I still studying homeopathic theory and attending seminars on new remedies or new information about old remedies? Surely what would really pay dividends would be to improve the way I took a history from my patients. But how?

I started to notice even more carefully how the different homeopaths I had observed conversed with their patients. I ignored what I did not like and modelled what I found useful. As I've mentioned before, there is hardly any useful literature on the subject. So how could I learn more?

I realised that at the heart of the homeopathic conversation was the doctor–patient or homeopath-patient relationship. Rapport was everything.

Six years at medical school had taught me nothing about it. The various homeopathic teachers, apart from Dr Ledermann, had not said much about it, so I had to look elsewhere to improve what I had increasingly begun to see as the very essence of the homeopathic process.

I enrolled on a course in counselling, described in more detail in Chapter 9. It was one of the most useful courses I have ever attended. The patient-therapist relationship and trust was at the centre of it all and the exercises we were put through in that course had an immeasurably beneficial effect on my homeopathic consulting skills. In retrospect it was amazing that I was the only doctor on the course, especially as these skills were not part of any medical curriculum I had heard of. After this course I knew that the centre of my future homeopathic education would be all about learning to have better quality conversations with my patients. I now turned to the world of psychotherapy for inspiration but realised pretty quickly that I had to be selective in what I studied. Homeopaths do not have the luxury of meeting a patient one to five times a week for a few years before prescribing! However, psychotherapists are certainly interested in the relationship between themselves and their patients. Indeed, the conduct of the therapist in conversation with his client is considered to be of paramount importance.

I returned to Dr Ledermann with hundreds of questions about every 'psychobabble' word in the dictionary, such as projection, transference, counter-transference, libido, Oedipus complex and so on. He was mostly patient and kind but occasionally dismissive of ideas he did not admire. I began to realise that I was only at the fringe of a huge body of information and only a small percentage of it had any relevance to the homeopathic process. But the information that was relevant homeopathically was of enormous benefit to me. Not only did it improve my results in the clinic, but it made me more enthusiastic about being a homeopath. Above all, it made me finally appreciate the sheer elegance of the homeopathic conversation itself.

Chapter 3

Homeopathic Education

As has been mentioned there is very little literature on homeopathic history-taking or what is called, in European homeopathy, anamnesis. The existing literature comprises three main types of books:

• Materia medicae

• Repertories: books and computer programmes

• Books on homeopathic theory.

It is important to examine this literature as it contains the main body of information from which students are taught homeopathy.

Materia medicae

There are hundreds of books containing an enormous amount of extremely useful information on the homeopathic remedies themselves. Additionally, in recent times, comprehensive computer software programmes have become available. In fact there is so much information that the beginner homeopath often feels intimidated by the sheer volume of it all. Exceptional people have been able to learn by heart religious texts like the Bible and the Koran, but no homeopath has been able to memorise Allen's *Encyclopedia*[8] or Hering's *Guiding Symptoms*.[9] Nevertheless these books are reference works that no serious homeopath can do without.

There are abbreviated materia medicae, like Allen's *Keynotes and Characteristics*,[10] which are shorter but still very difficult to memorise. Then there are more 'user-friendly' books giving short descriptions of homeopathic remedies that are of some use to the general public in self-prescribing for acute conditions but of little interest to the serious homeopathic student. Thus there is no lack of information on the homeopathic remedies themselves. And if this isn't intimidating enough, there are new remedies being added all the time. In addition, the remedies we have had since the 19th century are necessarily reinterpreted by every new generation of homeopaths.

The best modern books on the remedies are those where the author bases his description of a particular remedy on what he has personally found to be reliable in his own experience. George Vithoulkas' opus, *Materia Medica Viva*,[11] a mammoth work in progress, is a good example of this. Unfortunately many authors have written books in which they simply restate what other homeopaths have written without clinical confirmation from their own practice. This is dangerous, as symptoms and keynotes of remedies tend to get spuriously reinforced by repetition in the literature.

The original materia medica was, of course, the provings themselves. In these early clinical trials of natural substances, Hahnemann and others self-administered pharmacologically active doses of many different substances, then carefully recorded the symptoms that resulted in a materia medica. These are well described in Hahnemann's *Materia Medica Pura*[12] and Hughes' *A Cyclopedia of Drug Pathogenesy*,[13] neither of which are hardly read at all by modern homeopathic students. I recently picked up one of the four volumes of the latter and read the proving of the remedy, Platina. I doubt that many experienced homeopaths would be able to identify this remedy from reading its proving alone. The modern drug picture of Platina is just so different from its proving. What happened was that the homeopaths over the years have added clinical symptoms to the description in the materia medica. A clinical symptom is one that does not appear in the provings but has been added by homeopaths who have agreed on its reliability from their own clinical experience.

The addition of these clinical symptoms to the materia medica was perhaps the cause of the great rift between British and American homeopathy in the late 19th century. British homeopaths like Hughes and Dudgeon were reluctant to include them in the materia medica as they realised that adding these clinical symptoms was hardly a scientific process. Allen's *Encyclopedia*[14] was originally intended to be a transatlantic co-operation between Hughes and Allen but Hughes pulled out because he thought that Allen was too casual about what information he wanted to include.

Kent and the other Swedenborg-influenced American homeopaths went even further. Kent started to describe the remedies in the form of drug pictures that were both much easier to digest and included a huge amount of information based on his own clinical experience and that of his colleagues. Other American homeopaths such as Nash, Farrington and many others did the same thing. It is a small tragedy for homeopathy that it is now difficult to distinguish between clinical symptoms and those that appear in the provings. At one time it would have been possible to mark the clinical symptoms with an asterisk but that opportunity has now been lost.

What is important to know is that the Americans won the dispute very easily. The works of British authors such as Hughes and Dudgeon, who insisted on sticking with only those symptoms that appeared in the provings, are hardly read at all these days by homeopathic students while books such as Kent's *Lectures on Materia Medica*[15] have become classics. I believe this happened simply because the American homeopaths were getting much better results, especially with chronic diseases.

Perhaps there is a simple explanation for this. The original provings were one of the most noble and exciting medical experiments ever undertaken. This is even more evident when one considers the awful medicine that was being practised at the time. (This included bloodletting, leeches, emetics, purgatives and agents provoking salivation, perspiration and urination.) Nevertheless they were undertaken by a very small number of provers, many of whom were fairly insensitive to the remedy. Therefore it was inevitable that the information from these provings would be incomplete. They were indispensable as skeletal structure to the picture of a remedy but the flesh had to be added by clinical experience. In my opinion, Kent and his colleagues were victorious because they were astute observers of what sort of patients responded to the remedies they tried. They then started to include certain features of these patients directly into the materia medica. Therefore we learn that being female and having blonde hair and blue eyes give you a better chance of responding to Pulsatilla and being fair, fat and flabby makes you a candidate for Calcarea carbonica. However, it is pretty clear that if you fed a brunette with brown eyes Pulsatilla in any potency for any number of years she would not turn into a blue-eyed blonde! Nevertheless it is quite possible that people with pale skin and red hair may have a better than average chance of being successfully treated with Phosphorus. In fact the homeopathic literature is full of information that could not possibly have originated from the provings. The term 'classical homeopathy' might not even have come into being had it not been for the inclusion of these clinical symptoms. The simple fact is that almost all the materia medicae studied by modern homeopathic students include these clinical symptoms, and without them we would never have the drug pictures so vividly described by Kent, Tyler and many others.

Modern classical homeopathy relies heavily on these drug pictures which are as much descriptions of types of people as lists of symptoms. The descriptions of these types of people can be quite subtle and that is why it is so important to take good histories from your patients. As an effective classical homeopath you need to match detailed descriptions of drug 'types' to subtle information from your patients. If you are unable to elicit this information you may still get results from keynote prescribing but you will often miss the remedy because you never really understood your patient.

If homeopathy was the simple but difficult process of matching the symptoms of the patient to the symptoms that appear in the provings, we would not need to be so proficient at taking a good history. But the classical homeopath of today does not operate this way. His goal is to record all the physical and mental symptoms of his patient and, following the instructions of Hahnemann, to rate the psychological symptoms more highly than the physical. In the homeopathy of today, this often means matching psychological profiles of patients to psychological profiles of remedies. Although this may seem straightforward to begin with, it is far from easy to get reliable results in the clinic doing so. In homeopathy as in everything else, the proof of the pudding is in the eating. This process is made even more difficult by the fact that the drug pictures are not static 'photographs' of patients. They are more like movies of a person's life. That is why it is much harder to treat chronic disease than it is to treat acute problems with homeopathy.

The acute picture of the remedy Arsenicum album is very clear. It includes vomiting, diarrhoea, fearfulness, restlessness and collapse. In other words it resembles the symptoms produced by a person poisoned by a large dose of arsenic. This is well described by Flaubert in the death of Madame Bovary. If we see an acutely ill patient with some of these symptoms we can confidently prescribe Arsenicum album. However the chronic picture of Arsenicum album probably resembles what could happen to a person if a very small (but tangible) amount of arsenic were added to their evening meal for a few years. We would observe a gradual production of symptoms over a long period of time, eventually causing death. The psychological profile of this patient would go through many changes over the years. Thus if we consider this changing picture as a movie, we will have many different photographs of the remedy Arsenicum album. Thus Arsenicum album may be prescribed for a patient who is overly fastidious and a bit restless (resembling an early stage of the poisoning) or a patient who is dying in great fear and anguish (the late stage of the poisoning).

If we wish to match our patients to the complex, changing physical and psychological profiles that appear in the materia medicae in current use, we need to elicit some very subtle information about our patients' whole lives, past and present.

Modern technology has the capacity to revolutionise the materia medica. Many homeopaths all over the world have been recording their consultations on video for teaching purposes for quite a few years now. Soon all video recordings will be digitised. It is clearly possible to create a digitised live materia medica. Experienced homeopaths all over the world could be encouraged to collect cases on video where the constitutional remedy has clearly acted. With the patient's permission, of course, a small segment of the consultation would be selected. This may be a highly significant moment in the conversation or simply three or four minutes' recording of the patient talking about anything at all; his job, the weather or the day's news. It would depend totally on what the patient would allow the world homeopathic community to see. Most patients who have been helped significantly by accurate homeopathic prescriptions would co-operate.

The homeopath could then e-mail this small segment of the consultation to the person compiling this live materia medica. This segment of Ignatia, for example, would then be put on a DVD together with other successfully treated Ignatia patients and slowly and surely a remarkable materia medica would emerge. The homeopathic student, after reading a description of the remedy in an orthodox materia medica, would be able to put the DVD into his computer, click on that remedy and see a succession of short clips from videos of patients successfully treated with that remedy. The homeopath would not be listening for specific facts. The aim would be to absorb, both consciously and subliminally, the feel of the different presentations of that remedy. Therefore the language spoken by the patient would not be that important. After many years of homeopathic practice we do learn to recognise a few patients' remedies almost as they walk into the room. This is intuition based on experience of seeing many other patients respond to the remedy needed by the patient in front of us. Some homeopaths call these medicines 'favourite remedies' but they are just remedies they know well and recognise in patients. This type of materia medica would be a big step in sharing that type of recognition. Science fiction? I think not. The only impediment to creating such a materia medica would be the patient's legal position. This could be solved relatively easily by getting them to sign a form giving permission for the author to use a specific video clip.

Either the patient's homeopath or the collator of this digital materia medica could simply get them to fill out a legal form of consent for this via electronic mail. I feel this is an idea whose time has come and would provide an exponential increase in the prescribing skills of homeopaths everywhere. It would be a way of sharing our 'favourite' homeopathic remedies with the whole international community of homeopaths for the benefit of all our patients. A study of these video clips would also encourage homeopaths to develop their observational skills while listening to their patients.

Repertories

The history of the use of repertories in homeopathy is a fascinating subject. Suffice to say that Hahnemann apparently had his own personal one which he did not publish, Boenninghausen published the first comprehensive repertory and Kent wrote the most useful one. I consider Kent's repertory to be one of the most remarkable books ever written. The work that must have gone into producing any single page of it is almost unimaginable. His *Lectures on Homoeopathic Philosophy*[16] may have influenced many classical homeopaths; the publication of his *Lectures on Materia Medica*[17] was probably the birth of what we now call classical homeopathy; but Kent's *Repertory of the Homoeopathic Materia Medica*[18] was a contribution to homeopathy of unparalleled significance.

This magnificent book gave countless homeopaths the luxury of looking up in a single volume those symptoms of their patients they considered important. It simply recorded comprehensive materia medicae like the 12 volumes of Hering's *The Guiding Symptoms of Our Materia Medica*[19] in a different, but incredibly useful, way. Instead of listing symptoms under the heading of a remedy, we are now able to look up a symptom and see what remedies are associated with it. And not only that. We are also able to assess the relative importance of a remedy listed under that symptom. It also allows the cross-referencing of a number of symptoms commonly referred to as repertorisation. For this opus alone, James Tyler Kent deserves homeopathic immortality and he has every chance of acquiring it. His repertory has made life immeasurably easier for countless homeopaths. Without repertories we would have to memorise huge tracts of the materia medica and hope to remember them in relation to any given patient! Even more important is the benefit to homeopathic patients. We, classical homeopaths, must acknowledge a huge debt to Kent because we are all aware of how many times his repertory has helped us find the effective remedy.

In recent times Kent's repertory has been added to and changed, especially after it became available as computer software. There is a danger in adding information in an indiscriminate way but as long as the additions and changes are carefully marked and attributed to their authors, the usefulness of the book should be increased rather than diminished by these additions.

If we, as homeopaths, did not have repertories we would have to spend many decades on the intensive study of the materia medica. We still need to study materia medicae for reasons of speed in choosing a remedy before or after repertorisation but repertorisation will often produce some remedies we would not have thought of or might not even have heard of. Then we can simply compare the drug picture of that remedy with the information we have obtained from the patient. The repertory, whether in print or on a computer, is indispensable in homeopathic case analysis. It is an invaluable link between the information gained from the case history and the materia medica.

However, it is still the responsibility of the homeopath to choose what symptoms to repertorise. If the wrong information is selected, the repertory will very efficiently select the wrong remedy or group of remedies. For repertories on disc, the famous computer mnemonic GIGO is apposite – Garbage In Garbage Out. As wonderful a tool as it is, the repertory can do nothing to compensate for poor history taking. If the case has been taken well, the repertory can help even the beginner homeopath come up with a list of remedies containing the simillimum or a remedy that will be clinically effective. If the case-taking has not elicited the essential information from the patient, repertories, computers and materia medicae will prove to be useless. The conversations we have with our patients are clearly the most important part of homeopathic medicine.

Books on homeopathic theory

The third category of homeopathic literature is composed of books on the theory and practice of homeopathic medicine. The most important book by far in this rubric is obviously Hahnemann's *Organon*, one of the most important medical textbooks ever written and *the* book on homeopathic theory. This is a book every homeopath must read at regular intervals in his career. Each reading will bring new insights to the reader and renew his interest in homeopathy. There are some beautiful-looking new translations of the *Organon* but, for me, Robert Dudgeon's revised translation (1893) of the 5th edition is a classic.[20] It remains available in an inexpensive paperback addition which incorporates William Boericke's translation of the 6th edition as a footnote wherever the 6th edition differs from the 5th. This makes it possible to read the 5th and 6th editions simultaneously, and this is exactly how the *Organon* should be read for very good reason.

It is vital to know what changes Hahnemann made to the 5th edition and for the student homeopath to be aware that the 19th century homeopaths on both sides of the Atlantic did not have access to the 6th edition. The works of Kent (*Lectures on Homoeopathic Philosophy*[21] is particularly important in this regard) and others are based on the 5th edition. This is why you do not read about Kent and his colleagues prescribing LM potencies. These only appeared in the 6th edition (§270) which was published 78 years after Hahnemann's death. It had been finished by Hahnemann in 1844 but kept unpublished by various members of his family until it was finally acquired by Hahnemann's biographer, Richard Haehl, in 1920. William Boericke, who helped Haehl recover the text from Hahnemann's descendants, published an English translation of the 6th edition of the *Organon* in 1922.

It is important to ask ourselves why Hahnemann revised his central text five times. It is not unreasonable to assume that he made changes as he learned more and more from clinical experience. If he had lived even longer than his 89 years he may well have revised it many more times. That is why I sometimes feel uncomfortable when homeopaths quote Hahnemann chapter and verse apparently to settle a dispute with a colleague. The *Organon* is not a religious book. It is a magnificent medical text, epoch-making in its time and unlike any other medical books of that era, highly relevant nearly 200 years later. But it was a work in progress in its time and had Hahnemann lived through the age of microbiology and the genome, I feel sure the *Organon* would have been revised appropriately. Therefore it is reasonable for homeopaths all over the world to share their views on the modern theory and practice of homeopathy.

By his own admission, Hahnemann does not say a great deal about the process of taking the case.

> This individualising examination of a case of disease, for which I will only give in this place, general directions
>
> *(Organon §83)*

Nevertheless he devotes paragraphs 83 to 99 to the homeopathic interview and gives a lot of valuable advice which will be referred to later.

There are many other books on homeopathic theory of which Hahnemann's *Chronic Diseases*[22] and *Lesser Writings*[23] and Kent's *Lectures on Homoeopathic Philosophy*[24] have had a huge influence on the way homeopathy has been practised for more than 150 years. Books have been written on the practice of homeopathy from Hahnemann's time until the present day. Most of these books discuss: how to analyse the case; prescribe the first remedy; what potencies to use; how to assess the effect of the remedy; the second prescription; homeopathic aggravations and so on. Some of these books have a few paragraphs on the homeopathic consultation itself but most concern themselves with the work that has to be done after the conversation with the patient. The homeopath–patient relationship has not been written about in much detail and this is regrettable. It would have been illuminating to know at least something about the difference in the style of case-taking between the American, Kent, and the Englishman, Clarke, for example. I would love to know more about how all the famous classical homeopaths of the past conversed with their patients.

Books on homeopathic theory will continue to be written for many years. They would be very much improved if every author spoke openly about their conversations with patients, significant moments in the consultation and both appropriate and inappropriate interventions by themselves in the process. The quality of our consultations differs from day to day and from patient to patient. We can learn a great deal from what we do well in the consulting room as well as from our errors. If we are prepared to share this knowledge it can be of enormous value to other homeopaths and homeopathic students.

Chapter 4

Taking the Acute Case

This book is mainly about taking the case of chronically ill patients with particular regard to the process of eliciting mental symptoms which are vital to accurate homeopathic prescribing. The detailed physical information needed by the homeopath in both acute and chronic cases has been well documented by many other authors. In fact it is probably best described by Hahnemann in paragraphs 86 to 89 of the *Organon* and the important footnotes that accompany them. Kent is also meticulous in making it very clear what sort of physical signs and symptoms the homeopath needs take note of in his monograph, *What the Doctor Needs to Know in Order to Make a Successful Prescription.*[25] Nevertheless I will discuss the taking of the acute case briefly, with emphasis on the all-important psychological symptoms.

Acute cases

Acute diseases, left untreated, are generally either cured by the body's natural defences or result in death or severe destruction such as in the case of polio. The aim of a homeopathic prescription in acute disease is:

• To make the first possibility, cure, the most likely outcome

• To expedite cure (in self-limiting diseases like the common cold).

For practical purposes there are two categories of acute cases:

• Patients consulting you for the first time

• Patients who have seen you before.

Patients consulting you for the first time

Here the homeopath is presented with a 'snapshot' of what the patient is like when he is ill. He should allow the patient to describe how he feels in his own words in the usual homeopathic way before asking any questions. After this it will be necessary to ask many questions about the modalities of the symptoms. This is because these patients, usually having seen only orthodox doctors in the past, have been 'educated' into thinking that these details are irrelevant to the doctor and even a waste of his time.

After noting all the physical symptoms and their modalities comes the important task of acquiring symptoms concerning the patient's mental state. All classical homeopaths know the mental symptoms to be of the utmost importance in both acute and chronic cases. In acute cases we are particularly interested in how the patient's mental demeanour or affect has *changed* since he became ill.

Unfortunately in cases we are seeing for the first time, we do not know what our patient is like when he is well. We can ask him simply how he feels about being ill but it is always useful to ask relatives how his behaviour and mood have changed since becoming sick. I have found that relatives tend to be very forthcoming when asked this question and to volunteer valuable information of which the patient may be completely unaware, embarrassed to speak about, or consider unimportant. In taking the case of a baby or child it is, of course, vital to speak to the parents but I have found that even very young children have been able to furnish me with useful psychological details about their ill parent. And they love to be asked to help with the case!

If you can find even a single, vital, psychological symptom that the patient has only experienced since falling ill, it can often lead you to the right remedy by simply cross-referencing it with the relevant physical symptoms and modalities. This is why homeopaths agree that acute prescribing is a lot simpler than treating chronic disease.

It is important to find out whether your patients have used homeopathy before and what remedies have apparently helped them in similar situations. They may well have prescribed for themselves or been given a remedy by another homeopath. A telephone call to that homeopath can often save you a lot of time if patients do not remember or were not told what remedy was given.

The hierarchy of information in homeopathy usually has strange, rare and peculiar symptoms at the top of the list, followed by mental and emotional symptoms. However, in the clinic, I feel that the very highest indication for prescribing a homeopathic remedy for any patient is the knowledge that a particular remedy has worked well for that patient in the past.

As a beginner homeopath in the early 1980s, I saw an elderly woman who was suffering from chronic hoarseness. I was taught by ear, nose and throat surgeons (ENTs) at medical school to take chronic hoarseness seriously and should regard it as 'cancer until proved otherwise'. Fortunately she had been fully investigated and told that 'there was nothing wrong with her'. I am always a little amused when doctors tell patients that there is nothing wrong with them. Why would a sane or even an insane person consult a doctor if there was 'nothing wrong with them'? What doctors mean when they say this is: 'We cannot detect any abnormality in this patient with the clinical skills and investigations at our disposal at this juncture in the history of conventional medicine.' Anyway, all the tests had failed to show anything pathological in her larynx and no treatment was offered, so she had decided to try homeopathy. (Homeopaths have been known to refer to such people as 'TEETH' patients, TEETH being a mnemonic for 'Tried Everything Else, Try Homeopathy'.)

I took her case, prescribed a remedy and the hoarseness went away in less than a month. In fact I only saw her twice at that time. About eight years later I was no longer working at that practice in Buckinghamshire but the patient came to see me in London. Her hoarseness had finally returned. Unfortunately for me I no longer had her notes. I had left them at the clinic in Buckinghamshire in the care of another doctor and for complicated reasons these notes had been lost by that clinic. I couldn't for the life of me remember what remedy I had given her! So, sadly, I had no choice but to retake the case. I ended up prescribing Causticum but a month later there was no improvement at all. At this point I sent her to a voice clinic in which she was examined by an ENT surgeon, osteopath and psychotherapist. Again nothing was found and I was actually told that the problem was 'psychological' with a poor prognosis.

I became determined to find out what my previous prescription had been. I remembered that when I worked in that clinic I used to ask a certain homeopathic pharmacy to send the remedies to my patients as there was no homeopathic dispensary in the area. 'Eight years ago, you must be joking!' he said when I phoned him but he promised to look at his records and see what he could do. A week later he phoned me. I had prescribed Phosphorus 1M. I asked him to send her another dose which was immediately effective. She has to date needed only four doses of Phosphorus 1M in well over 15 years now and it has always worked beautifully. Poor prognosis indeed!

The lesson here is that it is worth moving heaven and earth to find out what remedies have worked well in the past. Sometimes other homeopaths can be a bit protective of their patients and their notes and do not readily give you this information, which can be equally useful in acute and chronic cases. If this happens ask your patient to find out for you and to remind their previous homeopath gently that it is a patient's right to know what medicines have been given to them. When other homeopaths ask you the same thing always be as helpful as possible. It may be painful to lose a patient where there has been a splendid result but we must always remember that in homeopathy, as in any form of medicine, the patient comes first.

Patients who have seen you before

Here you have the ability to assess how the patient's psychological state has changed since this recent illness. You are presented with a snapshot of the present psychological state and already have a brief movie of the patient's life in your head or in your notes. The distinguishing characteristics of the photograph in the context of the movie of the patient's life are the psychological (and physical) symptoms that will lead you to a successful homeopathic prescription.

If you are seeing a patient from whom you have taken a full homeopathic history before, you may know what remedy or remedies have helped him in similar acute illnesses in the past. You are strongly advised to study these remedies carefully in relation to the case, even if they are not obviously indicated by the symptoms of the current illness.

You may also have successfully prescribed a constitutional remedy for the patient in the past. This can help you manage the case in two possible ways.

The first possibility is to choose a remedy which is listed in the materia medica as being complementary to the patient's constitutional remedy. Two remedies that are considered complementary to each other means that homeopaths over the years have discovered through clinical experience that if one of the two has acted in a patient, the other may also be useful at some point in the patient's life. For example, if a patient's constitutional remedy has clearly been established as being Calcarea carbonica, the homeopath should certainly at least consider the prescription of Belladonna for that patient when he has a high temperature. This is because experience has taught us that Belladonna and Calcarea are complementary remedies. A common mistake among homeopathic students is to confuse a complementary remedy with a related remedy. Remedies that are related to each other are simply those remedies which have similar drug pictures. Causticum and Phosphorus are related remedies because their materia medica pictures have much in common. However they are certainly not complementary to each other and are almost never both needed in the same patient even over a lifetime.

The second advantage you have in prescribing for a patient you have seen before is simply to prescribe the constitutional remedy in any acute illness. This is based on the premise that you know that a particular remedy is capable of acting as a 'holistic stimulus' (this term was introduced to me by Dr Eric Ledermann) to better health in that particular patient. If it has already helped the patient in a general way it may well help him with any acute problem as well. Homeopaths who favour this way of treating acute illness tend to dissolve a few pillules of the constitutional remedy in a glass of water and invite the patient to sip it every hour or so. In my experience this is often a useful way of treating acute disease, especially when the acute remedy is not clearly evident but you know which remedy suits the patient's general constitution.

On the other hand this is no excuse for you to be lazy in your taking of the acute case, as the following example shows. A middle-aged female patient, whose constitutional remedy happened to be Veratrum album, presented to me with a fever and sore throat. Her symptoms also included bad breath and increased salivation. I examined her throat and saw a purulent, follicular tonsillitis on the right side. I took a swab of the tonsil and sent it to a laboratory for microscopy. I do remember a few things I learned at medical school! I then quite confidently prescribed the remedy, Mercurius iodatus flavus, which suited the acute symptoms and signs perfectly. The next day, the fever had subsided and the patient felt very much better in herself. A day later the tonsil no longer looked inflamed, merely slightly enlarged. I do not believe that a prescription of the constitutional remedy, Veratrum album, would have produced such a dramatic response. If the acute remedy is clear, as it was in this case, my first plan of action is to prescribe it in preference to the constitutional remedy.

It is wise to remember that seeing your patient when he is acutely ill can also help you find the constitutional remedy. Acute illness is a challenge to the whole organism and its immune system. How the person reacts psychologically to acute pain or discomfort is valuable information about the patient's constitution. Patients suffering from chronic problems tend to get used to their symptoms to some degree and unconsciously adapt their behaviour accordingly. When someone is acutely ill you are more likely to see the 'real person'. We consider it important to know whether a patient appreciates sympathy from others when he is feeling ill or when he has suffered some form of hardship. When taking the chronic case you might have to ask the patient this question directly or preferably ask the people he lives with. In an acute case it will generally be obvious to patient, family and homeopath whether the patient wants to be looked after or is 'aggravated by consolation'.

Patients tend to select their homeopaths carefully, often on personal recommendation. This is in distinct contrast to how they choose orthodox general practitioners, who are mainly selected on geographical location. This means that patients often live far away from their homeopaths. It is not uncommon for homeopaths to have patients who live in different cities and even countries from themselves.

Acute problems tend to happen out of surgery times and your initial contact with a patient of yours who is acutely ill is often on the telephone. This is a big problem as patients generally expect you to advise them homeopathically there and then. In cases where the patient has been treated successfully for exactly the same condition in the past and the condition is not potentially serious, you may recommend that they take the remedy that has acted in the previous episode, although I would advise you to be cautious in these cases and tell the patient or a family member to contact you if the condition does not improve quickly.

If a child has a fever, or an adult abdominal pain or the patient is suffering from an acute condition I have not treated before, I always insist on a physical examination. Ideally I would like to do this myself but this is not always possible for geographical reasons. However it is essential that this sort of patient is at least examined by a doctor, even if that doctor is not a homeopath. This is important for two reasons. The first is that it may be impossible to find the right homeopathic remedy over the phone. In the case mentioned earlier of tonsillitis treated with Mercurius iodatus flavus, it would have been very difficult to find that remedy without a physical examination. The second reason is much more serious. By prescribing over the telephone for an acute condition, you may obviate in the patient's mind the need for a physical examination. This can result in important orthodox medical diagnoses being missed. Neck stiffness and a rash are invisible on the phone and you only need to miss one case of meningitis to end your career or leave you feeling guilty and ashamed for life.

This leaves the problem of dealing with acutely ill patients whom you are unable to examine for the following reasons:

• Inability to come to your consulting rooms

• Unhappiness about the cost of a home visit

• Resistance to being seen by a doctor who is not a homeopath.

This is a problem that comes up almost every week in my own practice and I am sure is common in the practices of many other homeopaths. So how do you deal with it?

I end up having some interesting conversations over the telephone with my patients in these situations.

> *I am really sorry that I cannot recommend a homeopathic remedy this time, Mrs Brown. Although it is highly unlikely that your child has a serious illness like meningitis or pneumonia I cannot exclude that possibility over the phone and I can't take a chance with young Jonathan, not even if the chances are one in a thousand.*

If that does not convince her I may even say (with a reassuring laugh):

> *I can just see the judge saying: 'Dr Kaplan, this five-year-old child had a temperature of 40 degrees and you prescribed a homeopathic remedy over the telephone without even examining him!'*

When having these telephone conversations, it is important to remember that your patient is feeling unwell and is hardly in the best of spirits. He may also be an extremely anxious and sleep-deprived parent. Therefore it is necessary to be as warm, compassionate and reassuring as possible in these situations. The patient must be made aware that you are acting in the interest of his health or the health of his child. If the right tone is found, you will often find that the patient understands and appreciates this. You may even share a little laugh together if you exaggerate your own anxiety about missing a diagnosis and ending up in court!

When a patient is talking to you on the telephone he is usually in his own home or place of work. These are psychological environments where he feels more comfortable than when he is in your consulting room. He may well express himself differently, thus giving you useful information about himself.

Whenever you do not have direct access to your patients' files it is always worthwhile keeping a notebook handy to make notes which can then be added to the relevant file. I have stickyback labels near the telephone in my home. These can simply be stuck on to the latest page of the patient's notes and are often helpful when the patient next visits me in the surgery. Palmtops are also ideal for this purpose, and indispensable if your consultation notes are made directly on to a computer (an increasing tendency among homeopaths about which I have more to say in Chapter 17). It is then possible to download the information from your telephone call via the palmtop into your patient's file on your computer at work.

I have found both the palmtop computer and the mobile phone increasingly useful in my work. Of course, I am unavailable on the phone while consulting, unless it is a matter of life or death, but I don't mind taking brief calls from patients at most other times. Patients can be fearful or depressed when acutely ill and a few reassuring words can make all the difference to them. It is important not to speak for too long or you will find yourself conducting your whole practice on the telephone. The palmtop computer can easily store all your patient's telephone numbers, addresses and even remedies they have been prescribed. Soon they will be able to store all the patients' notes as well. It is also the diary of the future, allowing you to see any appointment you have made for the rest of your life. For those of you who prefer pen and paper, I apologise for ending this chapter on acute prescribing with 'techno-talk'. However, we are living in the 21st century.

Chapter 5

Approaching the Chronic Case

By far the majority of the consultations in my own practice are with people suffering from chronic disease. I am aware that this is not necessarily the case for all homeopaths but there are very few of us who will be able to avoid the challenge of the chronic case.

Hahnemann had tremendous success treating acute diseases, not least in the cholera epidemic of 1831.[26] It was homeopathy's success in the treatment of acute diseases that led to its rapid adoption by so many physicians all over Europe. It was only much later that Hahnemann started to address the problems of treating chronic disease. This led to the introduction of miasmatic theory into the *Organon* and the publication of *Chronic Diseases* in 1828.[27]

It is not my intention to discuss the theory and debates behind the treatment of chronic diseases. The aim of this book is to focus on the conversations homeopaths have with their patients in the hope of improving the art of taking the case. Nevertheless it is important to ask ourselves what exactly we are hoping to achieve during a consultation with a patient suffering from a chronic disease.

I consider myself to be a classical homeopath and in every chronic case my aim is to find the constitutional remedy of the patient. But even this needs clarification. What is a 'classical homeopath' and what is the 'constitutional remedy'? I have attended enough international homeopathic seminars and conferences to know that these terms mean different things to different homeopaths. They are far from easy to encapsulate in neat definitions so I will express what they mean to me. Below are listed a few of the features of my understanding of what is meant by these terms.

Classical homeopathy:

• Aims to find a single remedy at any given time in the case that will act as an holistic stimulus to the organism, prodding it towards health

- Includes the use of a Hahnemannian or more modern view of miasmatic theory
- Is respectful of Hering's law of cure
- Uses only one remedy at a time
- Puts a very high emphasis on the psychological and emotional symptoms of the patient.

The constitutional remedy can be defined as:

- A medicine that has clearly acted as a positive holistic stimulus in a patient, improving his health generally as well as giving at least some relief to his symptoms
- Often (but by no means always) selected on the totality of the patient's symptoms, both physical and psychological, but with greater emphasis on the psychological.

I have seen cases where the constitutional remedy was found via a single rare and peculiar symptom. In these cases the remedy did not match the totality of the rest of the symptoms particularly well but was not strongly contra-indicated either. An example of such a case from my practice was a 15-year-old boy who came with his mother to see me for a very severe rash on the soles of both feet. He had seen several dermatologists and used both antifungal and hydrocortisone creams. During the history he spoke very little and reacted to some homeopathic questions with disdain. Examination of his feet revealed an extensive, inflamed and scaly rash covering both soles. I had no other symptoms to go on so I simply consulted Kent's repertory and found the following rubric in the section, 'Extremities: Eruptions, desquamating, foot, sole of': there was only one remedy in italics and that was Mancinella. I then tried to 'elicit' some other Mancinella symptoms like 'fear of insanity' and 'fear of being taken by the devil'. If at first he had thought I was eccentric, he then looked at me as if I was stark, raving mad. With no other information to go on, I prescribed Mancinella 12CH with a superb result. A very good case to show to those people who believe homeopathic remedies to be placebos or that it is the homeopathic practitioner rather than the remedy that produces the result.

Other features of the constitutional remedy may include:

- A medicine that will help the patient on more than one occasion in his life (to distinguish it from nosodes used in the 'never well since an acute disease' situation which are also capable of acting as powerful holistic stimuli but seldom on more than one occasion in the same patient)

- Improving the patient's health by removing symptoms in the order of Hering's law of cure

- Improving the psychological wellbeing of the patient as well as relieving physical symptoms. This is confirmed when the patient reports that he 'feels better in himself'.

I don't expect you to concur totally with the ideas above but I hope that I can safely assume that we can all agree:

- That it is vital to record a full picture of as many as possible of the patient's symptoms, past and present as well as physical and psychological

- That an accurate assessment of the patient's psychological state is of the utmost importance in helping us find the constitutional remedy.

So how do we acquire this vital information?

I was taught to take the homeopathic history in a particular way and order. I see now that the purpose of this rather formal approach was to ensure that the homeopath does not omit to ask about certain vital areas of his patient's health. The following summary illustrates this approach.

- **History of the main complaint:** the patient initially is encouraged to describe his symptoms in his own words without interruption. When he has finished speaking he may be asked questions concerning modalities of the symptoms and the order in which they appeared

- **Other complaints:** the patient is asked if he has any other problems or symptoms and may be questioned about the modalities of these

- **Past medical history:** information about illnesses and signs and symptoms in the past. This is of particular relevance if they suffered from 'miasmatic' diseases such as gonorrhoea or tuberculosis or from any disease that seemed to initiate their present problem.

The topic of sexually transmitted diseases is hardly an easy subject of conversation with someone you have known for less than an hour. A patient consulting you for asthma, headaches or irritable bowel syndrome could well be shocked by a direct question about venereal disease. After all, what could an attack of gonorrhoea, successfully treated with a single injection of penicillin 30 years ago, have to do with his constipation? Miasmatic theory is not common knowledge and the patient may choose to keep such information to himself, depriving you of vital homeopathic clues. I get around this tricky issue by asking the following question:

> *Have you ever suffered from any infectious diseases such as rubella, typhoid, cholera, anthrax, yellow fever, gonorrhoea, syphilis, NSU (non-specific urethritis), tickbite fever, tuberculosis?*

This obviates the need to ask a direct question about sexually transmitted diseases and gives the patient the chance to deny the whole list. However he also has the opportunity to pick out an infectious disease he has suffered from in the past. In this way you will have given him the message that it is important for you to know about such illnesses. He may choose to be honest there and then but if he is embarrassed to speak about such things at the first interview, he may decide to return to this area in a later appointment.

- **Past surgical history:** why and when any operations were performed

- **Medications:** past and present, orthodox, homeopathic and other 'alternative' medicines.

- **Vaccinations:** especially if there was any reaction to the vaccination or if the present illness dates back to a vaccination

- **Systematic history:** open-ended questions are asked about any possible symptoms in all the organ systems (cardiovascular, respiratory, gastrointestinal, endocrinological, neurological, urogenital, dermatological and so on, covering the functioning of every organ in the body)

- **Generals:**
Reactions and general preferences regarding:

  1. *temperature*

  2. *climate*

  3. *geographical location*

  4. *time of day*

The patient's relationship with food:

1. *strong cravings*

2. *strong aversions*

3. *time/s of the day when most hungry*

4. *disorders produced by specific foods.*

Sleep:

1. *position while sleeping*

2. *snoring*

3. *unhealthy waking times (eg, 2 or 3am or regularly interrupted sleep)*

4. *depth of sleep*

5. *dreams, especially recurrent dreams.*

- **Mentals:** the patient is asked to describe his personality in general terms. When he has finished speaking, open-ended questions may be asked about anxiety, fears and phobias, emotional states, jealousy and envy, reactions to sympathy, sexuality, ability to express emotions like grief and anger and any aspect of the patient's psyche and personality both of the past and present.

I was taught that unsolicited symptoms were of greater value than answers to direct questions and was advised not to interrupt the patient.

> Every interruption breaks the train of thought of the narrators, and all they would have said at first does not again occur to them in precisely the same manner after that.
>
> *(Organon: footnote to §84)*

This is as true today as it was in Hahnemann's time when the patient is describing his symptoms or personality. If you interrupt a patient when he is talking about himself he may unconsciously feel rejected in relation to that particular topic and never speak about it as openly as he was before the interruption. It is interesting to note that this is entirely consistent with Freud's view of communication with patients, but of course this was a century before the time of Freud.

However, as Hahnemann notes: 'and refrains from interrupting them unless they wander off to other matters' (§84). If the occasional interruption was needed in Hahnemann's time, it may be even more necessary today. This is because most of the patients we see today have been seen by other doctors and been investigated and 'diagnosed'. They have also usually read articles in newspapers and popular magazines about their disease. An increasing number of my patients have studied their illness with the aid of a search engine on the internet. In fact there are many websites on the internet aimed at exactly such patients. The ability to gain information about disease on the internet is likely to increase as the internet becomes more and more an integral part of life in this century. Patients may feel empowered by this access to information and being able to break into the previously 'closed shop' of the world of medicine, but it is far from useful to the homeopaths taking their cases.

Information acquired by patients about their illness may not help you find their remedy but is not without its uses. I always thank patients for any information they have printed out from their 'research' on the internet. Doctors and homeopaths today have to live with the fact that many patients will know more about their particular disease than any professional who is not an expert on that particular illness. It is best not to be threatened by this. Data about the patient's orthodox diagnosis are useful in that it keeps us informed about the natural history and prognosis of that particular illness. Any medical textbook on your shelf is likely to be less up-to-date than information brought to you by your patients.

Some patients have presented me with whole books about their illness. These books can be useful, bland or dogmatic about a certain alternative way of treating a certain illness. I have a policy of accepting all such books with thanks and a promise to look at them later. Any apparent rejection of the book could be detrimental in creating rapport. How long I spend reading these books in my own time is up to me and obviously depends on my assessment of the book.

When patients educate themselves in these ways about their disease it has an important bearing on classical homeopathic case-taking. Instead of innocently describing his subjective experience of his disease which means relating his symptoms, he may use the jargon of modern, conventional medicine. When this happens it is sometimes advisable to make a timely and polite interruption. This is illustrated by the following example which is hypothetical but very typical of how many patients speak as they begin to tell me why they have come to see me.

Homeopath: *(after a friendly introduction) So, tell me what brings you...*

Patient: *Well, my general practitioner sent me to the hospital where they did a gastroscopy but they didn't find an ulcer. The gastroenterologist said that there was some inflammation and that I had a small hiatus hernia. The blood tests...*

Homeopath: *(interrupting gently) I am sorry to interrupt you but can I ask you what you felt when you first became ill rather than what doctors have told you? Perhaps you can start with when you were last well and tell me what happened to you.*

Patient: *(often looking quite relieved) Well about three years ago I woke up in the middle of the night with this terrible burning pain in my stomach.*

Homeopath: *(says nothing but relaxes into his chair, non-verbally communicating that he is interested and has plenty of time to hear the whole story.)*

The key to making a useful interruption of this kind is in your tone of voice. If you sound impatient, pushy or irritated you will have damaged your case-taking, sometimes irreparably. But if you use a gentle, reassuring and warm voice as you speak, you can get away with this sort of interruption and save a lot of valuable time. Of course it is not enough only to sound reassuring, warm and caring, you actually have to be reassuring, warm and caring!

Your patient, having received the message that you are more interested in his experience of his illness than what the doctors have told him or what he has read, may feel an enormous sense of relief. After all he is much more at home in the world of his own symptoms and feelings than in the world of medical jargon.

The approach of classical homeopathic history taking is very respectful of the patient's feelings and the patient senses this. We try to make the homeopathic case-taking as patient-led as possible. This is a major difference between the homeopathic approach and the way I was taught to take a standard medical history. I was encouraged to be courteous to patients and to try and develop a good bedside manner, even to allow the patient to tell his story in his own words. The medical approach, however, is to listen for vital clues that will lead us to a conventional diagnosis. You might listen politely as the patient talks about his emotions, fears and relationships. However, as this information is relatively unimportant in arriving at a diagnosis, the quality of listening will be quite different from that of the homeopath who must listen not only to every word but also to the tone of voice in which it is expressed. This is the beauty of homeopathy. The content of what the patient says is important but the way it is presented to us is at least of equal value.

Good homeopathic case-taking values everything the patient says and the way the conversation between homeopath and patient evolves is led by the patient, in contrast to a conventional case-taking which is very much led by the doctor. The homeopathic history is totally inclusive of a competent, orthodox, medical history but also covers a great deal of other territory. The classical homeopath is obliged to listen carefully to every word uttered by his patient. This is exactly what makes our profession special. The undivided attention of the homeopath to his patient creates an atmosphere in the room in which the patient feels respected, understood and even loved. This is the elegance of the homeopathic conversation.

It was this special feeling about the atmosphere of the consultation, conveyed to me by that very first book on homeopathy that I read all those years ago in Johannesburg, that was largely responsible for me choosing to specialise in homeopathic medicine. As a beginner, I experienced very little of this atmosphere as I rather rigidly stuck to the 'questionnaire' style of taking the case. Later, after observing many expert homeopaths in action and 'feeling' the atmosphere they created in their consulting rooms, I began to adopt a looser and more relaxed approach. I started to experience very short moments of a special quality that I could not name. I know this now simply as a feeling of 'forgetting oneself'. In these moments your patient feels totally received and invited to trust you and tell you exactly what his real 'dis-ease' is. Eighteen years later these moments are much more frequent but by no means consistent. It probably takes the better part of a lifetime to master the art of the homeopathic conversation. But there are some things in life that are worth waiting for.

As an orthodox medical doctor, I could look forward to retirement at the age of 65. As a homeopathic physician, I now hope to achieve consistency in competent case-taking by then! In orthodox medicine you are considered over the hill at that age. The profession feels that it's time for new blood. In homeopathy we may only reach our prime in our sixties. It's good to have something to look forward to as we age and homeopathic wisdom appeals to me more than growing roses. It is not surprising that homeopaths seldom retire before the age of 80 and many continue well beyond that.

Much of the rest of this book is about creating that special psychological atmosphere in your consulting room in which your patient feels invited to give you that intimate information about himself which is the essence of his problem or exactly where his 'dis-ease' is. You can only invite your patient to trust you enough to do this. He may have conscious or unconscious reasons for not doing so and we must respect this too and wait patiently for months on end in the hope that one day he will feel the time is right for him to tell us what is really the matter with him.

One of the most important and simple things I have learned about talking to patients is to be much more flexible in the order in which things are done and questions are asked before and during the homeopathic consultation.

When I first began taking homeopathic cases I stuck carefully to the order of that table shown earlier. This was because I wanted to ensure that I did not forget to ask the patient important homeopathic questions. This has the small advantage of being comprehensive but this is outweighed by the big disadvantage of making the patient feel as if he is being interviewed according to a rigid questionnaire. I now know that in the first interview, the creation of rapport between patient and doctor is far more important than ensuring that I have recorded every detail of the patient's story.

Here is a brief description of the way I now acquire homeopathic information from my patients. This is just a style that suits me at the present time. It may or may not suit you so I suggest that you take from it only what feels right for you.

Before the consultation

If you make your own appointments on the telephone you will get useful information from the patient there and then. This is valuable material as your potential patient is on familiar ground in his own home and does not dream that the homeopathic consultation has already begun! Tone of voice, background noise or voices of relatives may all give valuable clues.

If you have a receptionist who makes your appointments, ask him to make a note of any patients who sound peculiar or distinctive in any way. I have found all receptionists happy to oblige in this way and it tends to make them feel much more creative in their work. It never ceases to astonish me how certain people behave so well in the consulting room and yet I am constantly told by my receptionists that they are abusive and rude to them on the telephone and even in the waiting room. In other words this sort of patient is putting on a bit of an act or wearing a mask while talking to me but revealing an aspect of his real self to the receptionists. A brief, daily chat with the person who makes your appointments can yield surprisingly useful homeopathic information.

Bringing the patient to the consulting room

Some doctors and homeopaths speak to their receptionist on the phone and ask for the patient to be sent to the consulting room. I don't think that this is a good idea and I escort my patients to the consulting room, at least for the first visit. I begin by introducing myself with a genuine smile and always offer to shake their hand unless the patient is a woman dressed in the garb of a religion that forbids any unnecessary physical contact between a man and a woman who are not married to each other. For example an orthodox Jewish woman may be recognised by a head-covering (scarf, hat or wig) and concealing clothes. It is also useful to know that an orthodox Jewish woman is forbidden from touching or sitting too close to her husband or any man during her menstrual cycle.

If I see that the patient has a companion I make it clear immediately that I have no objection to that person attending the consultation. The choice is theirs. Even as we walk towards my room I find something to chat about, such as how they first heard of me. If they are carrying a book I generally ask them about it. This may lead to another topic of conversation and I have sometimes chatted to a patient for two or three minutes before asking them why they have come to see me. This is simply to create rapport and is by no means always appropriate. I simply do what feels right in the moment. On reaching the consulting room I offer to hang their coats up and use a wooden hanger of the very best quality for this purpose. I then ask them to make themselves comfortable.

A recent example from my own practice showed me just how important this pre-consultation period is. A new patient was booked in for 3pm. For some reason I only managed to go and fetch him at 3.12pm. I knew that I was exactly 12 minutes late since I felt a little guilty at the time, as I have learnt that time boundaries are very important. As I shook the patient's hand I noticed that he was a determined looking, middle-aged man wearing a smart leather jacket and obviously very angry about something. I guessed it might be that he had been kept waiting but made an instant and conscious decision not to apologise.

As I started to take his name, address and occupation (business tycoon) he could restrain himself no longer and told me how much he hated being kept waiting. He had made a long journey to see me and managed to be punctual, so the least I could do was to be there on time myself. As he spoke I could feel the atmosphere in the room become very energised. Nevertheless, on this occasion, although I realised that I was being provoked, I was able to remain calm and apologise, explaining that sometimes doctors have emergency cases. He seemed unimpressed and said: 'Okay, but I just had to say that!' He might as well have had the words 'Nux vomica' tattooed on his forehead. I took the case in the normal way and was not surprised that his main complaint was a problem with digestion, that he was an ex-alcoholic and now functioned well as a high-powered businessman. Many other symptoms confirmed the diagnosis and on seeing him a month later it was clear that the remedy had definitely acted. A clear case of Nux vomica before even starting to take the case! Sometimes homeopathy is delightfully easy. But not often.

Starting to take the case

When the patient has settled down I ask him for his name, address, contact telephone numbers, date of birth, marital status (including ages and names of children) and occupation. I like to chat a little about the patient's work. This is a topic about which he is used to talking about so it is a good way of breaking the ice. In normal conversation with people we have just met, work is often the first subject we discuss. If we want the homeopathic conversation to be as natural as possible it is quite reasonable to spend a minute or two on what the patient does every working day.

History of the main complaint

Finally I ask the question 'What brings you here today?' or sometimes 'How can I help?' This is a key moment in the consultation. The patient may unconsciously be deciding whether you are a person he can trust enough to have an authentic conversation with. You have little control over this decision. I just try to relax and 'be myself' in the hope that if he senses that I am not wearing a mask, he may choose not to wear one himself.

Now comes a time to listen. This listening is not a passive process, however. Your patient will be acutely aware of your interest in his story or when your attention wanders. What goes on inside the head of the homeopath during the interview is of paramount importance and we will return to this subject in Chapter 9.

An interruption is only necessary if the patient wanders off into the medical jargon, as I mentioned earlier. Otherwise this is a time for active listening, careful observation of the patient and good eye contact.

'Anything else?'

When the patient has finished speaking, I wait for a while before using the famous question, 'Anything else?' or 'Is there anything else you would like to say?' This phrase has been recommended to homeopaths with good reason.

It is a neutral, non-leading prod allowing the patient to feel comfortable in continuing to talk about himself. However I seldom use it more than twice in the consultation. Otherwise I start feeling like a parrot and who wants to confide in a parrot?

Details of the main complaint

When the patient has finished talking spontaneously and is not responding to my gentle verbal nudges to continue, I ask some questions about the various symptoms they will have mentioned. Questions about details of the main complaint will sound natural to him. In fact this is the moment where he may begin to notice the difference between a homeopathic and conventional medical consultation. As I ask questions about the modalities of the main complaint he will realise that I am interested in the minutiae of his subjective experience of his illness. This will hopefully make him feel that he and his illness are being equally respected.

Finally, when I feel satisfied that I have recorded as many modalities of the main complaint as possible, I prepare myself psychologically to ask a very revealing question.

'How does that leave you feeling?'

'That' is the most striking symptom they have mentioned so far. For example, a patient consults me complaining of recurrent migraine headaches. After listening to a detailed description of the pain I ask the relevant questions about modalities and find out that the headaches occur approximately every ten days, last 36 hours, are aggravated by noise, occur mostly in the area of the right temple and feel 'like toothache'. When I am satisfied that I am not going to get any more useful modalities I initiate the following type of dialogue.

Homeopath: *Can you tell me how the headaches leave you feeling?*

Patient: *The pain is very severe and I can't do much.*

Homeopath: *Well, actually, I was thinking of how they affect your mood.*

Patient: *I'm not very happy when I have them!*

Homeopath: *What do you mean by 'not very happy'?*

Patient: *What do you mean?*

Homeopath: *I wondered what sort of emotions you are experiencing when you have the headaches.*

Patient: *I feel upset that I have a headache again.*

Homeopath: *Upset?*

Patient: *Yes, it's damn annoying to have these migraines. People who don't suffer from them haven't got a clue what you are talking about.*

Homeopath: *So you feel annoyed?*

Patient: *Yes, sometimes I feel very angry indeed but what can I do? The painkillers don't work and my doctor won't give me stronger ones because he says I will become addicted to them.*

Homeopath: *And when you are angry about having a headache, how does that anger leave you feeling?*

Patient: *Just angry, really angry.*

Homeopath: *About having a headache?*

Patient: *Well sometimes I feel angry about other things as well.*

Homeopath: *Like what?*

Patient: *I do so much for my family but when I have a headache, nobody seems to care much. Perhaps it's because they are used to me having headaches, but that doesn't help me!*

Homeopath: *And how does that make you feel?*

What this example shows is a relatively seamless transition from discussing the main complaint to talking about the person himself or the 'mentals'. The patient expects to be asked about the main symptom they are presenting. They may be a little surprised at all the modalities you ask about, but they tend to appreciate the attention to detail. Then it is quite natural to ask them how the symptom leaves them feeling emotionally.

After learning something about how the patient feels emotionally while they are experiencing any symptom, it feels quite reasonable to ask about that emotion in general terms. Suddenly you are talking about the inner feelings of the patient and it does not seem very strange to the patient at all.

Other methods of taking the case may move from the main complaint to 'other complaints' but I feel that it is more natural to move from the history of the main complaint to the 'mental symptoms' in the way I have illustrated. Some patients may not need as much prompting as in the example used. As soon as they are asked about how the pain leaves them feeling they may go into a short monologue which should not be interrupted under any circumstances as these are reliable psychological, homeopathic symptoms which will be very valuable when analysing the case.

If you choose to move from the main complaint to an area other than the psychological symptoms, eventually you will need to ask a direct question about their personality. I have heard homeopaths say things like: 'In homeopathy we are interested in the whole patient as well as the problem so I would like to ask you some questions about your personality' This often results in that bemused expression on the face of the patient that is familiar to all homeopaths.

On reflection it is not unreasonable for a patient suffering from a very painful ingrown toenail to be surprised when asked to describe his personality or whether he has any fears and phobias. He may well be thinking: 'What possible relevance can this intimate information be to my ingrown toenail? Why is the doctor asking these strange questions about my private life?' And in a worst possible scenario: 'Is he some sort of voyeur?'

It is worth comparing this method of asking about the mental symptoms to the following type of dialogue.

Homeopath: *And when your toe is really hurting how does the pain leave you feeling?*

Patient: *I feel terrible. I just can't do anything and I have so much to do and the antibiotics have been no help at all. The doctor says I may need to have surgery and I really don't want to have an operation.*

Homeopath: *Why not?*

Patient: *Well (with a sad expression) when I was a child my best friend had an operation and…*

And now you have effortlessly and naturally moved the conversation into the psychological realm and it feels fine for homeopath and patient to stay there for a while. And the most useful question which achieves such a transition from the main complaint to the mentals is:

And how does the pain (or any symptom) leave you feeling?

Then it feels natural to prompt the patient into talking about other areas of his personality like fears and phobias and their emotional life in general. Of course the conversation at this level requires considerable skill. This is what most of the rest of this book is about. Talking to patients has been correctly described as the *art* of homeopathy by George Vithoulkas (in conversation) while study of materia medica, case analysis and the conducting of provings may be considered the science of homeopathy.

The order that I acquire information in the consulting room varies according to each patient but can be represented as follows:

• The history of the main complaint and its modalities

• The question: And how does the symptom leave you feeling?

• A natural follow-up question regarding 'feelings'

• A natural transition into the rest of the mentals

• All other homeopathic questions except the generals

• The generals.

After talking about the patient's feelings and personality, I feel free to ask about anything except the generals. These I leave until last. This is because factors such as temperature preferences and food aversions and desires tend to prejudice me in favour of certain remedies which I then find hard to get out of my mind. It is preferable first to hear about the suppressed grief of a Natrum muriaticum case and only later have the diagnosis confirmed by learning that they have a craving for salt. If I learn about a patient's craving for salt at an early stage my mind becomes prejudiced in favour of remedies such as Natrum muriaticum, Phosphorus, Veratrum album and others whether I am conscious of this prejudice or not.

> This individualising examination of a case of disease…
> demands of the physician nothing but *freedom from prejudice*…
> *(Organon §83)*

The italics in the above are Hahnemann's and we will return to discuss the term 'freedom from prejudice' in another context.

Chapter 6

Receiving Vital Information

There is a tendency in the current practice of classical homeopathy to focus strongly on the mental symptoms. Several modern materia medicae (Zaren[28], Bailey,[29] Coulter[30]) describe only the psychological profile of various remedies. This, not unreasonably, assumes that the reader is familiar with the physical keynotes or that he can easily learn them from any number of other textbooks. This is indicative of the swing towards the classical approach in homeopathy which now seems to be an international phenomenon.

This does not mean that other methods of prescribing are ineffective. On the contrary, the following three ways of analysing the case can often yield a remedy that has a profound effect on the whole organism:

- Keynotes
- 'Never well since an acute illness' syndrome
- Causation.

Keynotes

A prescription based on three or more good keynotes can often be clinically effective. Books like Allen's *Keynotes and Characteristics with Comparisons*[31] have not become classics without reason. The problem for the homeopath is that it is very difficult to get good keynotes from your case-taking. Sometimes you hear what sounds like a good keynote symptom but it does not appear in the repertory or materia medica and therefore cannot help you prescribe a remedy. Keynote prescribing may be appropriate for the general practitioner who is interested in homeopathy and is able to recognise a keynote symptom when he hears one. For the professional homeopath it is insufficient in itself as a strategy for effective prescribing.

'Never well since an acute illness' prescription

Patients who have been unwell in some way since an acute illness may respond to a nosode of that disease. Personally I have found this method of prescribing very unrewarding except in cases of tuberculosis, syphilis and gonorrhoea where it can be very effective indeed – whether the remedy fits the rest of the case or not.

I remember a case of a neatly dressed gentleman with an arthritic problem whom I saw many years ago. The case looked like a very clear case of Arsenicum album. I confidently gave the remedy in a high potency and was most disappointed when on the second consultation he reported no improvement. I was at a loss as Arsenicum still appeared to be the remedy that fitted the totality of his symptoms. Under 'Past Medical History' (PMH) I noticed that he had suffered from tuberculosis as a child. Nothing else in the case suggested a prescription of Tuberculinum but having run out of ideas, I prescribed a single dose of Tuberculinum 200CH. The result was dramatic. I wondered afterwards if he then would respond better to Arsenicum album but I have never prescribed it for him, preferring to repeat the Tuberculinum which has been necessary only twice in ten years. It is wise to remember that the highest indication for a remedy is that it has worked well in the patient in the past.

Causation

This sort of prescription is based purely on the collective experience of homeopaths over many years. Examples include:

• Any problem dating since an injury – Arnica

• Mental symptoms dating back to a head injury – Natrum sulphuricum (I have had some excellent results prescribing Natrum sulphuricum on this indication alone)

• Ailments dating back to a vaccination: Thuja, Vaccininum and others (see the rubric Vaccinosis in the Generals section of the repertory).

There is part of the Mind section of the repertory called 'Ailments from' which lists certain causative factors of illness and the remedies to consider in these cases. There is also a large section, called 'Causation' in Clarke's *Clinical Repertory to the Dictionary of Materia Medica*[32] which complements his *Dictionary of Practical Materia Medica.*[33] Of course the prognosis is much better if the remedy that suits the causative factor also suits the patient overall.

Prescribing on causation can be easy and rewarding. Our problem again is that these cases constitute a very small minority of the patients we see.

The modern, classical homeopath knows that an understanding of the psyche of his patient is of paramount importance. If physical keynotes are present, they are useful but he cannot rely on eliciting them from his patient. Most case-taking does not produce them. If a clear causative factor can be found it is invaluable, but this is relatively uncommon. Therefore we must rely on the advice of Hahnemann and base most of our prescriptions on the totality of the patient's symptoms. Hahnemann also recommends a hierarchy of symptoms with mental symptoms at the top.

> This holds good to such an extent, that the state of the disposition of the patient often chiefly determines the selection of the homeopathic remedy, as being a decidedly characteristic symptom which can least of all remain concealed from the accurately observing physician.
>
> *(Organon §211)*

In other words, the psychological features which determine the 'disposition' are considered the most important individualising information in determining the constitution of the patient. But this alone is not a good enough case for giving such a high priority to the mental symptoms in homeopathy. We still need medicines that have these mental characteristics as part of their drug pictures. In the very next paragraph, Hahnemann assures us that such medicines do indeed exist.

> The Creator of therapeutic agents has also had particular regard to this main feature of all diseases, the altered state of the disposition and mind, for there is no powerful medicinal substance in the world which does not very notably alter the state of the disposition and mind in the healthy individual who tests it, and every medicine does so in a different manner.
>
> *(Organon §212)*

So the modern, classical homeopath is fully justified in spending plenty of time in trying to determine the 'altered state of the disposition and mind'. In taking the case of a chronic disease we have little idea when this alteration first took place. Of course if the patient (or a close relative) tells you that his personality has changed since he became ill, then the ways in which it has changed will comprise the essential symptoms which we use to make a prescription. However, we do not usually hear this and must use any psychological symptoms present in the patient to give ourselves a picture of his 'disposition'.

The classical homeopath thus needs to know the inner man, his most intimate psychological weaknesses – that part of the patient that is most vulnerable and therefore most protected. It may be so vulnerable that the patient will often wear a mask so the world does not see it. Obviously this is no easy task. If your patient has spent a lifetime hiding it from the world, perhaps consciously, but more often unconsciously, why should he suddenly reveal it to you?

We often, quite irrationally, hope to acquire this information simply by asking our patient to describe his personality. Direct questions about various facets of his personality such as fear, anxiety, jealousy and envy are even less productive. Why should he suddenly trust you enough to reveal to you his most intimate fears and neuroses? Who are you after all? A 'homeopath' who has been recommended by a friend; mentioned by his general practitioner; picked at random from a list of homeopaths; or found in the Yellow Pages after a lonely, desperate, search for help when all else has failed. Why should he trust you with information that hardly seems relevant to his main complaint?

So how are we to get this essential information about the psyche of the patient? Let us turn once again to the *Organon* and see if Hahnemann can help us.

> After this is done, the physician should endeavour in repeated conversations
> with the patient to trace the picture of his disease as completely as possible
> *(Organon §209)*

The clue is in the phrase 'repeated conversations'. By saying this, Hahnemann makes it clear that he is aware how difficult it is to get the facts we need from our patients. How many conversations are implied by 'repeated'? Two, three, four or more? Is it just possible that Hahnemann suggests that we keep conversing with the patient until he trusts us enough to give us all the information we need to make a confident prescription?

Some years ago I thought that the ideal way of practising homeopathy would be to see patients weekly for a one-hour conversation until I had a strong feeling that I understood the case reasonably well and could begin to think of making a prescription. I asked myself what I would want if I put myself in my patient's shoes. Would I want my homeopath to be obliged to prescribe after the first consultation, whether he felt confident about his prescription or not? Or would I prefer to come back for 'repeated conversations' until he intuitively felt the time had come to give me a remedy? This is a rhetorical question for anyone who knows the power of the simillimum. But there are practical difficulties in doing this. Patients can be suspicious. After all, their general practitioner might only spend seven-and-a-half minutes with them so it may be difficult for them to understand why a homeopath needs so much of their time.

So far I have been unable to practise the homeopathy of 'repeated conversations'. Of course we all have repeated conversations with our patients. The difference is that we tend to prescribe a remedy after each conversation. If I feel that I don't have enough information after the first visit, I no longer feel obliged to analyse the case and make a speculative prescription. I tell the patient that I feel we need to talk more and ask him to return for another hour of conversation. If he is unwilling to do so, I regard it as his problem and not mine. As I have said, I have no doubt whatsoever what I would want for myself were I the patient and my homeopath said the same thing to me. However, after the second hour, I do feel under pressure to prescribe a remedy. I look forward to the day when I will have the confidence to follow Hahnemann's advice to the letter and insist on as many conversations it takes to leave me feeling relaxed and confident about my prescription.

But I can hear you asking: 'Aren't "repeated conversations" a great luxury?'

Well, it all depends what you compare homeopathy to. If you compare it to the work of a general practitioner and the number of patients he sees in a day and the amount of time he spends with them, then yes, it's a huge luxury. But if you compare it with the work of a psychoanalyst who sees a patient for nearly an hour – the famous '50-minute hour' – three to five times a week for several years, then it is no luxury at all. The average psychotherapist or counsellor might see a patient for an hour once a week. A course of psychotherapy comprising ten such hours is called 'brief therapy'. In most situations the therapist would prefer many more sessions. It is not at all uncommon for a patient to see a psychotherapist for several years.

A general practitioner may see 200 patients a week, a psychotherapist 25 and a psychoanalyst eight. Where do we homeopaths fit in? We have established that intimate, protected, psychological information is usually the key to a successful prescription. And yet we compare ourselves much more with the medical model than with the model of psychotherapy. It seems illogical. We are interested in both physical and psychological information about our patients but we value the psychological more highly. Surely we have more to learn from those practitioners who routinely have the 'repeated conversations' recommended by Hahnemann with their patients?

Chapter 7

Influences

'Sitting in' with experienced homeopaths is a time-honoured method of learning classical homeopathy. When I first started sitting in with colleagues and teachers, I was mainly interested in how they analysed the case, what remedies they chose, why they chose them and in what potency they prescribed them. It soon became clear that homeopaths had quite different styles of taking the case and this aspect of homeopathy began to be of great interest to me. I watched some colleagues use more or less the same method of interviewing in every case whereas others seemed to change their style from patient to patient. Some homeopaths seemed to chat in a friendly way with patients while others seemed to remain silent most of the time. Some had fairly serious conversations and others had a more light-hearted approach and shared the occasional joke with the patient.

Homeopathic interviews also differed from homeopath to homeopath with regard to the actual questions asked, how they were asked and the order in which they were asked. I became fascinated by the different types of conversations I was observing. Different types of conversations between people represent different types of relationships. I realise now that this was the start of my interest in the relationship between homeopath and patient. If I sat in on a single interview I was able to observe only a snapshot of this relationship. Even such a glimpse was of great interest to me but I realised that for a deeper understanding it would be necessary to sit in on a series of consultations between the same homeopath and patient. This is far from easy to do. Unless I sat in with the same homeopath every day for a few months, I was not going to be able to see many homeopath-patient relationships in progress. I wanted to see the 'movie' of the relationship rather than just the occasional 'photograph'.

In 1982 I sat in with the same homeopathic doctor, Dr Eric Ledermann, every Thursday afternoon for the whole year. Inevitably I began to see some of the patients return for follow-up visits and to observe continuity in their management. Dr Ledermann is a homeopath but he is also a practising psychiatrist and psychotherapist. Obviously I was only allowed to attend his homeopathic clinic. After a patient had left the consulting room, we not only discussed the homeopathic management, but often spoke about what had transpired in the room and our general feelings about the patient. We analysed the conversation that had just taken place between the patient and Dr Ledermann and even how that conversation had left us feeling. Initially I was only interested in the homeopathic interpretation and management but I was not to be let off the hook so lightly.

I remember a case of a young boy with a skin problem who came in with his mother. When he told us he was seven years old, Dr Ledermann smiled benignly and joked about him getting old. We all laughed and the rest of the interview went smoothly. As soon as he and his mother left, I was asked what I thought about the consultation. I said that I thought that it had gone fairly well and started to talk about possible remedies. However my teacher was not interested in talking about homeopathy this time. 'No', he said, 'I should not have made that joke about him getting old. I realised after making it that he was too young to hear something like that and it might have left him feeling confused.' This was a remarkable moment for me. An experienced homeopath and doctor over the age of 70 had chosen to be critical about himself in regard to a particular moment in a consultation. In fact it had left him feeling uncomfortable, even a little guilty, and as far as I had been concerned the consultation had been uneventful. He had obviously paid a lot more attention to the doctor-patient relationship at the time than I had.

We began to talk about the various types of relationships that occurred in different forms of medicine. These included relationships between doctor and patient, homeopath and patient and psychotherapist and patient. In his case these were all happening simultaneously in many cases. He did not feel obliged to prescribe a remedy or even 'think homeopathically' every time. What was always stressed was what had happened between doctor and patient. This was quite a new way of analysing the case! And a very valid one.

In my basic homeopathic training I had been taught by Dr Charles Kennedy (a former president of the Liga Homeopathica Medicorum Internationalis) that the feelings of the homeopath in the consultation could occasionally be useful. The example given was that of a child in pain. If you felt sorry for the child and wanted to pat its head, I was taught, the most likely remedy was Pulsatilla. However if you felt that you wanted to slap the child in irritation the remedy was much more likely to be Chamomilla. In other words the feelings of the homeopath were occasionally useful diagnostically. However, this was the only example I remember being taught of how to use my own feelings as diagnostic tool. Now I had seen an experienced homeopath, doctor and psychiatrist be openly critical of his taking of a case. Each case would teach him more but he would never totally master the art of talking to patients. None of us ever will, but that is irrelevant. What is important is that we realise that there is always room for improvement in this, the most important part of the homeopathic process.

Sitting in on that consultation was a milestone in my career as a doctor and homeopath. From then on my thoughts and emotions during every consultation, as well as my actions, would be under surveillance whether I liked it or not. It would be many years later that I realised that the quality of my relationships with my patients was by far the most important factor in how successful I was as a homeopath and doctor.

This is not the case in every type of medicine. If you need a surgeon to perform a circumcision or an opthalmologist to fix your detached retina with a laser beam, a steady hand is of the essence rather than the rapport between patient and doctor. But in general practice, and particularly in homeopathy, the doctor-patient relationship is crucial. I could study the materia medica until remedies were coming out of my ears but if I was unable to create rapport with my patients, I might as well give up homeopathy and general practice and start studying surgery. So how was I to improve the quality of my relationships with my patients?

I was fortunate enough to have a mentor in this journey and that was Dr Ledermann. He had already written several books on holistic medicine, the philosophy of medicine and his own, unique brand of existential psychotherapy[34, 35, 36]. He had tirelessly trawled through the works of the classical philosophers such as Kant, the existential philosophers Kierkegaard and Sartre and the medical philosophers, in particular Jaspers. And now I made my way through his own books with the wonderful advantage of being able to quiz him about them every Thursday afternoon. I heard new words such as teleology, epistemology and phenomenology. I started to have a small understanding of the thoughts of Kant, Husserl, Heidigger, Buber, Emerson, Jaspers, William James and Krishnamurti. And those were just the philosophers.

There was also the whole world of psychology and psychotherapy, starting of course with Freud, but including Jung, Adler, Klein, and many others.

Of course my study of the works of these 'Great Thinkers' was amateurish to say the least. But I was not studying for a degree in philosophy. In some ways I wished I was. This, I thought, is what they should have taught me in medical school. It would have been wonderful to have studied these great thinkers in depth at a university but that was not going to happen. I was also reading these authors with a particular purpose in mind. I was not studying them to improve my intellect. I wanted them to help me become a better doctor and homeopath. My reading always scanned for what was applicable and useful in this regard. In short I was highly selective in what I read. I did not have unlimited time for a very exhaustive enquiry. After all I had a day job as a homeopathic doctor.

I was on a search to answer the sort of questions that I posed in the introduction. What was I doing with my life as a doctor and homeopath? And why? I started to think about the dictum 'Physician heal thyself'. (My patients had often reminded me of it whenever I had the misfortune of missing work through illness!) I read about the concept of the 'wounded healer' and found myself staring into a mirror.

I started with the classical philosophers and psychologists who had influenced Dr Ledermann before he went on to develop his own brand of existential psychotherapy; and I began to find my own influences as well. J. Krishnamurti was a big influence. So was the work of William Reich, the neo-Freudian, who had realised the importance of the body and its behaviour and language in the world of psychotherapy. This led me to his pupil, Alexander Lowen, and bioenergetics. Thinkers who wrote about the mind-body connection always drew my interest. Surely that was what classical homeopathy was all about?

The journey of exploration continued. Laing, Perls, Grof, Janov, Golas, Joy, le Shan, Milton Erickson and the neurolinguistic programming people all came into the picture. Nevertheless I remained loyal to the existential and profoundly loving approach of my mentor. His view was that human beings have a conscience (axiomatic) unless they are psychopaths. In neurotic patients it is the task of the psychotherapist to make the unconscious conscience of the patient, conscious. All the methodology and thoughts of people like Jung, Freud and Adler could be useful in understanding the challenges people had to face in learning to get in touch with their conscience and live according to it. Libido, archetypes and society could all represent such challenges but all these could be put to the sword if you were persistent in trying to live according to conscience. This is exactly what I had seen him do when he criticised his own comments to that seven-year-old. His conscience told him he'd made a mistake, he noted it and he would be unlikely to make the same mistake again. It was important to learn from the various medical philosophers and psychologists but the conscience of the patient himself was central.

Many years later I read a passage in the introduction to John Rowan's *The Transpersonal* that summarised perfectly what I had been seeking.

> From this well-established base psychotherapy arches out into space, and the other end of the bridge seems to be hidden in mist. What we are aiming at in therapy has been variously described: the healthy person; the whole person; the fully functioning person; self actualisation; individuation; making the unconscious conscious, and so on. The concepts are vague and very open-ended, and a long journey seems quite often to be involved; it is hard to know whether one has arrived at the end of it. As one reaches the end of one span of the bridge, more spans become visible, further along the bridge. People who have ventured out further along this bridge include the Jungians, the psychosynthesis people, the transpersonal people, the Osho people; some of the biofeedback people such as Maxwell Cade; some of the primal integration people; some of the holistic health people and so on. Nearly all of these are very cagey about talking of the other end of the bridge: come a little further, they say, and we shall find what we shall find.[37]

We classical homeopaths are nothing if we are not 'holistic health people'. A good doctor always is – whether he knows it or not.

Through all this I remained a homeopath. No other approach or therapy attracted me more than classical homeopathy. I preferred it to everything else as I loved the way it valued the patient's subjective experience of his illness above everything else. This, to me, represented a profound respect for the individual. The fact that a prescription of a medicine could be based purely on this subjective experience of disease (or dis-ease) was deeply moving to me and has remained so.

I read and re-read the *Organon* and then I read Kent's classic text on the practice of homeopathy, *Lectures on Homoeopathic Philosophy*.[38] Published in 1900, it has been an inspiration to many classical homeopaths for the duration of the 20th century and looks like remaining so for some time to come.

I have made it clear why I regard Kent's *Lectures on Materia Medica*[39] and his *Repertory*[40] as homeopathic masterpieces, but *Lectures on Homoeopathic Philosophy*[41] is different. In some ways it is a commentary on the *Organon* itself but it also contains much of Kent himself and in particular the influence on Kent of Emmanuel Swedenborg.

Swedenborg (1688–1772) was a scientist interested in mathematics, minerals, anatomy and physiology, but it is for his theological writings that he will be remembered. He annotated the Bible, attempting to show the deeper and more mystical significance of every verse. This is not the place for a discussion on his contribution to theology and I am not the author to do it. What is absolutely clear, however, is that Swedenborg had an enormous influence on the way many important American homeopaths thought and consequently how they practised homeopathy. Homeopaths influenced by Swedenborg include Boericke, Tafel, Hempel, Gram, Guernsey, Farrington and many others, but his influence on Kent was profound.

As one reads *Lectures on Homoeopathic Philosophy* one comes across terms which are not part of the general homeopathic lingo. A good example of such a term is 'simple substance', a phrase nowhere to be found in the *Organon*, but certainly known to Swedenborgians. Julian Winston, in his excellent book on the history of homeopathy, *The Faces of Homœopathy*, writes:

> It is with the work of Kent that we see the ultimate linking of the works of Swedenborg and Hahnemann, for both men thought of disease as a matter of the spirit – the *dynamis*.[42]

Although it is unknown when Kent became interested in the works of Swedenborg, we do know that in 1893 he was attending 'doctrinal' classes, and by 1896 he was infusing his lectures with Swedenborgian ideas. As Swedenborg's work was a commentary on the deeper meanings in the Bible, Kent's *Lectures on Homoeopathic Philosophy* was a commentary on the *Organon*, dissecting each paragraph and telling us how to understand the deeper meaning within – but seen through a Swedenborgian filter.

In the work of Hahnemann, Kent saw a complete set of correspondences with the work of Swedenborg. We can see this clearly, time and again, in his lectures as he discussed 'simple substance', 'will and understanding' and 'series and degrees' within homeopathic practice.

I found *Lectures on Homoeopathic Philosophy* useful in parts; the section on assessing the results of a homeopathic prescription is logical, practical and comprehensive. Kent's sheer zeal and enthusiasm for homeopathy is infectious but the book is also very hard to digest in places. In some ways it seems to be written for homeopaths who are familiar with the works of Swedenborg. As I have mentioned, many of the great American homeopaths were Swedenborgians. For them the book would be a smooth read as they were familiar with the works of both Hahnemann and Swedenborg. After reading the book a second time, I realised that to understand it any better I would have to study the works of Swedenborg. This was a problem for me because by doing so I would be entering the realm of a particular religion, which in this case would have been a mystical version of Christianity. The homeopathy of Hahnemann is for all creeds and religions and although Hahnemann was a Freemason for most of his life, he seems extremely careful not to associate the *Organon* with any particular religion.

> There is in the interior of man, nothing morbid that is curable and no invisible morbid alteration that is curable which does not make itself known to the accurately observing physician by means of morbid signs and symptoms – an arrangement in perfect conformity with the infinite goodness of the all-wise Preserver of human life.
>
> *(Organon §14)*

Thus it is clear that Hahnemann believed in a divinity; but by describing this divinity as 'the all-wise Preserver of human life', he ensures that no religion can claim this divinity as their own. Thus the *Organon*, although deistic, cannot be allied to any particular religion, making it acceptable to people of all faiths.

I was studying homeopathy, psychology and the philosophy of medicine all at the same time and practising homeopathy as well. It was a joyous time. At last I was getting the education I had always hankered after. It was unstructured but in no ways diminished by that. It is a privilege to be a picker and a chooser. After all, I had been through so many years of studying medicine only from the mechanistic perspective. I saw this period of my life as a completion of my basic training in medicine. No lists to be memorised and no examinations; and no teachers or lecturers except for one mentor and supervisor. It was a gloriously liberating exploration and I began to ponder some of the questions with which I started this book. For the first time I felt I had made the right choice in studying medicine and this in itself was very reassuring.

I was reading a lot of 'heavy' literature, but there was a mischievous part of me always on the lookout for the absurd and the ridiculous and I found plenty of this in my studies. I have always loved to laugh and took an interest in the alternative comedy scene in London. I realised that the best comedians were modern court jesters whose job it was not merely to make people laugh but also to hold up a mirror to their audiences. As my friend, the comedian Arnold Brown,[43] suggests, we need to 'try to find answers to all these questions. Questions like... Why are we here? Where are we going? Who is going with us? Are we coming back? And above all: Shall we be taking sandwiches?'

Years later, I would learn that humour could be very effective in the consulting room. When homeopath and patient laughed together, rapport between them had probably been attained.

I saw that homeopaths had much to learn from those who had spent their lives studying the relationship between the patient and the doctor or therapist. A lot of what I studied was interesting in its own right but had no direct application in homeopathy. However, along the way I acquired insights, skills and techniques that have been invaluable to me in the homeopathic consultation over the past two decades. If there is a raison d'être for this book, it is to share these with you.

Chapter 8

Learning from Other Disciplines

When homeopaths present cases to colleagues they include information acquired in different ways. These are some of the ways we get homeopathically useful facts about our patients:

1. The patient voluntarily gives information without being subjected to a direct question. These subjective, unsolicited symptoms are considered very important by the classical homeopath.

2. The patient's spouse or relative give their opinions on the patient's symptoms and character. Their feelings about the patient may be more objective than the patient's own remarks and can be very useful.

3. The homeopath uses his personal observations of the patient as symptoms eg, the dirty, smelly, unkempt Sulphur and the restless, anxious, miserly Arsenicum album.

4. The homeopath asks the patient direct questions. This is considered by most classical homeopaths to be the least desirable way of taking the case. Nevertheless I have seen superb homeopaths like George Vithoulkas make effective of use of direct questioning. Direct questions can be helpful when the homeopath is thinking seriously of prescribing from a short list of remedies arrived at after careful analysis of the case. At this late point in the homeopathic conversation, it is not unreasonable to ask the patient about certain symptoms that comprise the materia medica picture of each remedy.

Here is an example of a useful direct question. Let us suppose I am thinking seriously of prescribing the remedy, Natrum muriaticum, for a patient after three-quarters of an hour of taking the case. At this stage I might well ask a male patient the question:

At a urinal, are you able to pass urine if there are several other men present or do you sometimes have to use a cubicle?

If the patient is female I might say:

Say you are sitting with friends in someone's living room and the toilet was very close. Would you be able to pass urine easily if you knew everyone in the living room would be able to hear you?

The main point of asking direct questions such as these is that it is unlikely that you will obtain this vital piece of confirming information in any other way. If the patient confirms this symptom of being 'pee-shy' you have virtually sealed the case for Natrum muriaticum. If they do not, then you know you have more work to do.

5. The homeopath uses his own feelings as a barometer of what the patient is feeling. This is an uncommon way of assessing patients in homeopathy. The example of our inner reactions to the child needing Chamomilla compared with those towards the one needing Pulsatilla has been mentioned. Another example is feeling as if psychological barbs were being thrown at you, which is a 'symptom' of the patient who needs Nitric acid. I remember George Vithoulkas describing this particular feeling that homeopaths experience while in the company of Nitric acid patients.

6. The homeopath observes carefully how the patient is reacting to the homeopath himself. An example of this is the Nux vomica case from my own practice, described earlier, who was so furious when his consultation was delayed by 12 minutes. No homeopathic writer would ever advocate intentionally provoking our patients in this way but the observation of how my patient reacted to the provocation was far more useful in finding Nux vomica than anything obtained in the consultation itself.

It is common to hear about symptoms obtained by the first four means but unusual to hear about anything obtained from the last two. This implies that homeopaths are not overly concerned about acquiring symptoms from information directly connected to the actual relationship they have with their patients. The homeopathic materia medicae hardly describe these sort of data at all and yet the finest classical homeopaths of all time have always prescribed in this way.

A good example of such a prescriber was the late Dr Margerie Blackie, a very famous English homeopathic doctor and consultant at the Royal London Homoeopathic Hospital. I began my studies at The Faculty of

Homoeopathy soon after her death so I never had the chance of sitting in on her outpatient clinic. I have spoken, however, to many doctors who had seen her practise and all speak of her uncanny ability, often exercised, to decide on a patient's constitutional remedy minutes after the patient entered the room. The only way of doing this is to use non-verbal information (see Chapter 16). This may indeed include the use of visual clues but it surely also needs the homeopath to be sensitive to the inner, unspoken feelings of the patient and perhaps more importantly, sensitive to their own feelings which are either a reaction to what the patient is feeling or even the patients' feelings themselves which have been projected or displaced on to the homeopath. I feel sure that every 'gifted' homeopath is doing this and usually it is all happening at an unconscious level.

The process of prescribing like this is simple but by no means easy. You are listening to a patient complain to you that he is no better and you feel as if you are being attacked in some way. You then remember (perhaps unconsciously) that you experienced this very same specific feeling when talking to another patient in the past. That patient responded brilliantly to Nitric acid so perhaps this one is a case of Nitric acid as well. The confidence in using this feeling of being attacked as an indicator for Nitric acid grows as you experience the same feeling with a number of Nitric acid cases. Finally Nitric acid becomes one of your 'favourite remedies'. And therefore every homeopath has a different set of favourite remedies! A favourite remedy, in my opinion, is one which the homeopath is able to identify from non-verbal information based on the conscious or unconscious memory of previous cases treated successfully with that remedy.

As we gain experience by seeing more and more patients, the ability to assimilate non-verbal clues grows and so does the memory of successfully treated cases. This apparently makes us able to prescribe some remedies 'intuitively'. This is why I have advocated a modern, digitised, live materia medica on DVD. If after studying the drug picture of a patient in the materia medica, we then watch a series of very short video clips of patients who have been treated successfully by that remedy, we may well absorb this vital non-verbal information.

It is clear to me that the relationship we have with our patients contains incredibly useful information about the patient if only we knew how to access that information. Unfortunately very few homeopathic authors have explored this way of acquiring vital information about patients. Homeopathic writers may not have explored the value of looking carefully at their relationships with their patients as a means of enhancing the accuracy of their prescribing. But if homeopaths have not paid sufficient attention to this territory, other disciplines have. It is my strong belief that classical homeopaths have much to learn from these professionals and the way they relate to their patients.

We will now look at what well-known psychoanalysts, psychotherapists and counsellors have had to say about the therapist-patient relationship and the acquisition of useful information. Almost all of these authors have had much to say about the interpretation of this information, but that is not our concern as classical homeopaths. We have our own way of using the information obtained; so we will confine our exploration to only what is useful in the context of the homeopathic consultation.

Freud

We begin our exploration of such professionals by looking at the work of the father of psychoanalysis, Dr Sigmund Freud. Freud's contribution to our understanding of the unconscious mind and its effect on our lives is inestimable. It is owing to Freud that the following words and phrases have become significant in our understanding of the human condition: id, ego, superego; defence mechanisms; libido, penis envy, Oedipus complex; transference and counter-transference.

Our goal, however, is to look at only what is applicable to the homeopathic conversation. Freudian psychoanalysts gather information from their patients in three main ways.

• Free association

• Dreams

• Parapraxis (the 'Freudian slip').

Free association

In classical psychoanalysis, the client (or analysand) is requested to lie on a couch, out of sight of the psychoanalyst, and recount whatever thoughts, feelings or images are going on inside his head. The analyst may or may not choose to make a comment but will often remain silent for long periods. The idea is that the unconscious mind of the patient will make itself known through this process in a symbolic way. The analyst facilitates the client's understanding of what emerges during free association, giving him an increased appreciation of the enormous influence of the unconscious mind on daily life.

We do not have the time in homeopathy for free association and I don't think our patients would stand for it, let alone lie down for it, if we did. Nevertheless, Freud's idea of the relationship of free association and the unconscious mind can be extremely useful to all homeopaths.

Freudian psychoanalysts and analytic psychotherapists seldom interrupt their patients as this might inhibit the flow of information from the unconscious of the patient. A century before Freud, Hahnemann was advocating the same thing when he stressed that the patient should be allowed to tell his story in his own words without interruption, as I have discussed. An untimely interruption would break the flow of information from the unconscious mind of the patient and Hahnemann is aware of this, as is clear from the incredibly astute footnote to paragraph 84 of the *Organon* where he states that if a patient is interrupted he will never return to talking about that subject in exactly the same way. The flow from the unconscious has been interrupted and the patient may have many possible negative reactions to this interruption, not least of which would be the feeling of some form of rejection.

When we remain silent and let our patients speak, we are inviting a type of free association in the hope of understanding our patients' problems at the deepest psychological level. We can learn from Freud to be increasingly comfortable with silence in the consultation. If the patient stops talking and remains silent there is no need to feel uncomfortable as we often do when this occurs in normal social intercourse. We can calmly wait for the next topic our patient chooses to mention. Often this will be of significance. The key is in the state of mind of the homeopath. If the patient senses that he is trying his homeopath's patience, he will find something to say to please the homeopath. What is said under these circumstances is likely to be of little use to the homeopath. The information volunteered after a period of silence in which the homeopath has been passive, but totally aware and ready to receive, can be the key to the whole case.

I remember a case of a colleague, Dr Denis Somper, that illustrates this well. Dr Somper is a classical homeopathic physician and a gentleman of the 'old school'. He is a retiring and private man and can seldom be persuaded to teach, much to the disadvantage of many doctors studying homeopathy.

However I will always associate the word 'unsolicited' with him. Over and over he stressed the value of 'unsolicited' information from the patient over anything obtained by a direct question. A woman in acute pain had consulted him. He had asked her to describe the pain which she began to do. Eventually she remained silent. As is his custom, he remained comfortable in that silence and waited for the next 'unsolicited' symptom. The silence continued. Eventually the patient could take no more of it and thumping her fist on the desk she yelled at Dr Somper: 'Don't just sit there, do something!' Dr Somper's description of what he did will remain forever etched in my memory. 'I gave her Chamomilla and *it* did something!' This was unsolicited information of the highest order. The patient did not tell him that she had the symptom 'angry when in pain' – she demonstrated it right in front of him. And this would not have happened if he had spoken instead of remaining silent – even though he must have been aware that his patient was not exactly as comfortable with the silence as he was.

The ability to remain silent in consultation is a function of the ongoing psychological development of the homeopath. This is not a recommendation to embark on the long journey of psychoanalysis, though I do know of some homeopaths who have done exactly that. The more comfortable you feel with yourself the more comfortable you will feel in this period of silence. Practise this in any social situation. Whenever there is an 'uncomfortable silence' in any conversation, no matter how trivial, try to enjoy that silence or at least not to be intimidated by it. Try not to be the person who breaks the silence. After a while you may well find yourself actually enjoying these periods of silence and this will be invaluable in the homeopathic conversations you have with patients.

Sometimes I have watched patients go into a period of silence that seems meditative. Then they snap out of this trance-like state and say something fairly trivial. I may choose to ask the question: 'What were you thinking about then?' It might turn out to be something of direct homeopathic importance or a pointer to a part of the patient's life that is well worth further exploration in the consultation.

Dreams

Dreams are the royal road to the unconscious.[44]

The patient's dreams were of great importance to Freud and they were important to homeopaths before Freud was born. They were important to the ancient

Greek physicians or priests who practised medicine at the temple of Asclepios more than two millennia ago. Patients used to sleep on the steps of the temple on the night before they saw the priest. The next day they would relate their dreams to the priest who would interpret these dreams and use them as clues to finding out what the patient needed to do in order to regain his health.

Freud felt that when we dream, our defences relax and the unconscious mind is able to express memories and fears that are often deeply suppressed in normal waking life. Obviously the classical homeopath is interested in such revealing material.

At medical school I don't remember anyone ever saying anything about asking patients about their dreams. No homeopathic conversation, however, is complete without hearing about the patient's dreams. I consider any dream worthy of inclusion in the analysis of the case if:

• It is recurrent

• It has made a big impression on the patient.

Having decided that a particular dream is worthy of being included in your case analysis, there are three ways of using the dream as a 'symptom':

• Consult the repertory

• Attempt an interpretation of the dream

• Ask the patient to interpret the dream.

Consult the repertory
You look up the dream in the section on 'dreams' in the repertory. If the patient's dream is listed, it can be invaluable in case analysis, especially if it is an unusual dream.

I remember the case of a middle-aged woman who came to see me for 'swelling of the feet'. On examination her feet and ankles were oedematous but she had been fully investigated and she was not suffering from heart failure, liver disease or any other cause of pitting oedema. When I asked her about her dreams, she mentioned that she had a recurrent dream of herself flying. The repertory had only one remedy in italics for this dream and that was Apis mellifica. Apis is also a major remedy for fluid retention so the combination of these two symptoms already made a reasonable case for the remedy. After chatting to her for a little longer I could see that her personality was certainly not incompatible with the mentals of Apis. She was a busy, active person and could be jealous at times. She responded very well and I have not needed to give her any remedy but Apis. The dream of flying was the key symptom and a simple reference to Kent's repertory more or less solved the case.

Attempt an interpretation of the dream

Of course there is no need to do this if the dream appears in the repertory. It can be very frustrating if a dream is obviously an important aspect of the case but is not listed in the repertory. I feel that it is unwise to discard the dream from your analysis, especially as there are certain dreams that have well-established interpretations. These can be looked up in a number of books on dreams and assessed to see if the interpretation may just be applicable in the case at hand. If it seems applicable to your patient, it would seem logical to discuss with him the psychological issues suggested by the dream. This discussion may bring out some useful mental symptoms. Needless to say, such 'pop psychology' books on instant interpretation of dreams are treated with contempt by most professional psychologists. However we can share this fact with the patient and still discuss the interpretation in the book. I might say something like: 'Well, your dream does not seem to appear in the homeopathic books so let's see if this book, *10,000 Dreams Interpreted*[45] (little laugh if it feels appropriate) has anything to say about it.'

I then read the 'interpretation' to the patient. It does not really matter that these books are not likely to be consistently reliable. What is important is that whatever you read from the book to your patient about his dream is likely to produce some reaction or at least lead to a talk about the book's interpretation of the dream. It's only effect may be that you and your patient both laugh at what the book says but the homeopathic conversation will certainly be no worse off for that!

Ask the patient to interpret the dream

You can ask the patient what the dream means to him. This simple open-ended question can be most useful even if the dream does appear in the repertory. The patient's interpretation of the dream, the way it is related to you, or even his reluctance to do so, can all be helpful when it comes to analysing the case.

We cannot afford to ignore a patient's dreams. They give valuable information because they occur when the patient's guard is down and therefore give us information we would never get from the patient while he is awake. As Prospero, perhaps the most evolved character created by Shakespeare, muses at the end of *The Tempest*:

'We are such stuff as dreams are made of, and our little life is rounded with a sleep'[46]

Parapraxis (the 'Freudian slip')

Freud did not believe in accidents. If a patient is always late for his appointments or 'forgets' to keep the appointment at all, his unconscious may be trying to express something, perhaps aggression towards you, or maybe resistance to getting better. The classic Freudian 'slip of the tongue' is when the patient 'accidentally' uses a word which *sounds* similar to the word intended but is nonsensical in the context of the patient's sentence. More importantly it reveals something directly from the unconscious mind of the patient. If a patient, referring to a musical conversation, says 'his penis' instead of 'his piece', therefore, it might be time to talk about his sex life.

Freud believed these little accidents and mistakes in writing and speech to be caused by unconscious motivational forces. They are not infrequent in homeopathic conversations and when you hear one, you should certainly prick up your ears.

Freud's contribution to the understanding of the human condition through his emphasis on the unconscious mind is inestimable. The philosophy of dualism epitomised by Descartes' famous dictum: 'I think, therefore I am' had ushered in a long period where mechanistic thinking was achieving a great deal in the sciences, including medical science, but as DeWitt and Baldwin point out, this also had some serious drawbacks.

Because of this emphasis, however, the objective and materialistic side of life achieved a commanding lead over that of the subjective and non-conscious, and it was not until philosophers such as Kierkegaard and Husserl, writers such as Dostoevsky and Tolstoy, and clinicians such as Freud, Jung and Adler, that the subjective world began to be explored in terms more appropriate to its understanding.[47]

The key word here for me is 'subjective'. The symptoms a patient experiences collectively comprise his subjective experience of discomfort or pain. These subjective experiences, as related to us by our patients, form the basis of our homeopathic prescriptions.

It is interesting to note that another physician of Teutonic extraction, by the name of Samuel Hahnemann, was not only carefully listening to patients describing their subjective experience of their illnesses, but helping them with both physical and psychological problems with homeopathic remedies based on those very subjective experiences, a long time before Freud. The first edition of the *Organon* was published in 1810, more than a century before Freud published his paper on 'The Unconscious' in 1915.

Before we leave Freud it is necessary to say something of the relevance of his concepts of transference and counter-transference to the conversations homeopaths have with their patients.

Transference occurs when the analysand directs emotions towards the analyst (psychotherapist) which at a deep level, he feels towards a parent or parental figure. For Freud, transference was the key to progress in psychoanalysis and only by the expression of it could the patient's problems be understood and resolved. Counter-transference occurs when the psychoanalyst (or psychotherapist) unconsciously allows responses to his patient to be governed by his own emotional conflicts, traumas and personal, psychological history. In everyday medical practice, this is often described as becoming 'too involved' with your patient. The Freudian therapist, having spent many years of his life in psychoanalysis and in 'training analysis' should try to avoid the expression of counter-transference which is counterproductive to the psychoanalytic process.

I have little doubt that both transference and counter-transference are regular features of many orthodox medical consultations and even more frequent in the more intimate environment of the homeopathic conversation. This is probably because homeopaths tend to spend an hour on the first consultation which is the usual length of time for a session of psychotherapy. In sitting in with other homeopaths, I have observed these processes in action on many occasions.

The expression of transference by the patient is as useful to the homeopath as it is to the psychoanalyst. An awareness of the nature of the transference may help the homeopath find a remedy indicated by deeply ingrained psychological traits. In the case mentioned earlier of the patient who was infuriated with me for being 12 minutes late, some knowledge of the concept of transference proved to be useful. I was aware at the time that his anger had less to do with my lack of punctuality than it had to do with some deep-seated anger towards a parent in the past. The anger itself was long-standing, deeply rooted in his psyche and spilling over towards me in freely expressed transference. This is typical of Nux vomica cases in my experience. As I have mentioned, the rest of the case history confirmed this remedy and he responded well.

The expression of counter-transference in homeopathic consultations is extremely common. This is because homeopaths do tend to get more 'involved' with their patients than conventional doctors do. The psychological boundary between patient and homeopath is more blurred than that between doctor and patient. This is because the homeopathic conversation inevitably and necessarily enters the area of the psyche.

I like the view expressed by Robin Shohet, an expert in the supervision of psychotherapists, that 'counter-transference is both inevitable and useful'.[48] This is somewhat antithetical to classical Freudian psychoanalytic theory. However it is entirely consistent with the recommendation in Chapter 7 to use the feelings that arise in relation to a patient as a diagnostic tool. As long as you are aware of the counter-transference in action, it can actually aid you in your search for that vital information about the psyche of the patient, which we classical homeopaths treasure so dearly.

Jung

Carl Gustav Jung, initially a devoted disciple of Freud, later fell out with his mentor. This was partially because he did not elevate sexuality to the same degree as Freud in the understanding of the psyche, but mainly because in describing the 'collective unconscious' he departed fundamentally from the Freudian viewpoint. He is also responsible for the terms 'introvert' and 'extrovert' ('open' and 'closed' personalities in colloquial homeopathy), 'archetype' and 'persona'.

It is not my intention to discuss these concepts because they are not directly related to the homeopathic conversation. However, homeopathy itself has been looked at from the Jungian point of view, particularly by Edward Whitmont who was an eminent Jungian analyst as well as a homeopath. In his book *Psyche and Substance*[49] different remedies can be seen as corresponding to the various archetypes.

As far as taking the case is concerned, Jung does not have much to add to what we have learned from Freud. A Jungian analysis would also use free association and dreams, though Jungians may analyse dreams in quite a different way from Freudians. When a patient's dream does not appear in the repertory and you are interested in what it means to the psychologists, you have the choice of Freudian, Jungian, existential and/or many other ways of interpretation. Personally I prefer to ask the patient for his own interpretation and take the discussion from there.

Voice Dialogue is an interesting, practical technique developed by Hal Stone,[50] initially a Jungian psychotherapist. It can fairly be described as a neo-Jungian form of psychotherapy. Stone postulates that we have various 'voices' in our heads such as 'the pusher'; 'the child'; the 'protector/controller'; 'the critic' and many others. Each 'voice' has something to say about its needs but in most of us some 'voices' tend to drown out the others. For example, the 'critic' may be shouting so loudly and censoriously about everything that the patient does, that the 'inner child' hardly ever gets a word in and the patient never really gives himself a chance to 'play'.

Stone's Voice Dialogue aims to give all the voices a chance to speak out and even to say what they think of each other. Two or more chairs are used and the client is asked to change chairs when it is time for a new voice to speak. This sort of dualogue is also used in Fritz Perl's Gestalt Therapy. The therapy is non-judgemental. It becomes clear to the client which voices are dominant and which are being suppressed. A healthy balance of the various voices indicates a healthy individual.

I mention Voice Dialogue as I have occasionally found a variation of it useful in the homeopathic consultation. I don't try to differentiate the typical voices when listening to a patient, but sometimes it becomes clear that there are two voices clearly in conflict with each other in the same patient. For example, a female patient was ambivalent about having the second child her partner was very keen on. In this situation two 'voices' were clear. There was 'a voice that wanted to have a baby' and one that did not. It was useful to separate these voices, simply by giving each a different chair. In this case 'the voice that wanted the baby' could speak of all the advantages of having another child. The patient was then asked to move to an adjacent chair and let 'the voice against having a baby' have its say as well as expressing its thoughts about the 'pro-baby voice'. Then back to the 'voice for', to hear what it thought about 'the voice opposing it'. On the few times I have used this, I have found that patients get the idea very quickly and even enjoy the process. It helps clarify things for both patient and homeopath and need only take 10 to 15 minutes of a homeopathic consultation.

After the duologue (I don't tend to work with more than two voices) the patient is brought back to a 'normal state' and asked what insights he or she might have gained from the process. It is often quite surprising what they can learn in such a short time. Of course any insights gained from the exercise, by either patient or homeopath, may prove to be of use when it comes to analysing the case.

This is a very unconventional way of taking a homeopathic history but it is my view that as long as the patient feels safe and protected and the homeopath is confident and skilled at what they are jointly doing, it is an acceptable way of gathering valuable homeopathic information. It can be regarded as a bonus if the patient is amused or helped by the little duologue and in my experience, this is often the case. A small word of warning here. For obvious reasons, this approach is highly inappropriate for patients with dissociative disorders or multiple personality disorders. These illnesses are rare and you would probably have noticed 'something strange' about your patient much earlier in the conversation and not even considered using such an avant-garde way of taking the history with them. In any case I would only recommend this sort of approach on the third or fourth visit, if the patient has failed to respond to remedies chosen and the normal conversation you are having with your patient does not appear to be yielding any new information. In addition, it should only be used by practitioners who have had some training in the technique and on patients with whom they feel safe.

Reich

Wilhelm Reich was a student of Freud but broke away from the mainstream to focus on studying the physical effects of repressed sexuality. He used massage and various forms of body work to release what he called 'muscular armouring', by which he meant the ways the body compensates and adapts to anxiety, fear and anger by, for example, tensing the muscles of the shoulder and neck when unable to express anger.

Different sorts of psychological tension and repression of emotions lead to various muscle groups becoming tense. This tension perverts the flow of energy in the body. Reich termed this energy 'orgone energy' and it has much in common with what Hahnemann called the 'vital force'.

Reich also believed that sexual orgasm can be an extremely healthy release of mental and physical energy. He called the capacity to achieve this psychological and physical surrender 'orgastic potency'. In his view, only a very small minority of people were able to experience this type of orgasm and release. Therefore most people are physically and mentally tense; an assertion that few physicians or psychologists would dispute.

Reich was ridiculed during his time and eventually imprisoned for his views but his work was refined and developed by people like Alexander Lowen in what he called 'bioenergetics'.

This particular tangent to psychoanalytic theory has something in common with homeopathy. Both are types of psychosomatic medicine. The homeopath and the practitioner of bioenergetics, or any Reichian-influenced psychotherapist, are interested in both the mental and physical symptoms of their patients. This leads to an attitude in the consulting room that is different from conventional medicine (mechanistic) and psychotherapy (psychological rather than physical), but includes features of each. The split between mind and body has been dispensed with and the human organism is considered to be animated by a vital force (homeopathy) or orgone energy (Reich). When this energy flows through the body and mind, unhindered by mental or physical obstacles, a state of health can be said to exist.

I have learned two things about homeopathic case-taking from Reich, Lowen and other types of 'bodywork' therapists.

First, muscular tension in the body is a valuable pointer to the psychological state of our patients. Sometimes they will tell you about their stiff neck and sometimes they won't. Sooner or later I examine this area in all my patients. They do not have to remove even a single garment. I simply ask permission to put my hands on their shoulders and examine that part of them. Tension, tenderness and painful 'nodules' in the area of the trapezius muscle usually indicates suppressed emotion, which is often anger. I have had many patients whose anger has only been admitted when I have felt this sort of muscular tension in their neck and shoulders and remarked on it. Obviously this has important ramifications on any homeopathic prescription that follows.

Secondly, the sexuality and sex life of the patient are vital topics of discussion in classical homeopathy. This is clearly evident from the materia medica and repertories which are full of sexual symptoms. The great homeopaths of the 19th century were living in fairly puritanical times and may well have been uncomfortable about the inclusion of so much sexual content in their books. They simply could not avoid facing the simple truth that sex is as important in homeopathy as it is in life in general.

There are many homeopaths who are embarrassed about asking patients about their sex lives. If you are one of them, it is important that you ask yourself why this is so. The good news is that it gets easier as you get older as an increasing number of your patients will be of a similar or younger age to yourself. As a male doctor, I have no problem in talking to other men about their sex lives. When it comes to female patients, I usually ask them about their menstrual periods and then ask: 'How is your sex drive?' This has the implication that I am just asking another question about their hormonal balance. You are more likely to get a straight answer if your tone of voice remains relaxed. The best way to sound relaxed is to be relaxed. Of course being relaxed when asking questions about sex depends on how comfortable you are with your own sexuality.

Asking questions about sex means asking about masturbation, which is a fairly taboo subject in Western society. This is quite strange as all the statistical surveys reveal that most people masturbate, whether they are single, married, heterosexual, homosexual or trans-sexual. What does the suppression of the sexual drive of the Conium maculatum patient actually mean? Is this someone who does not have sexual intercourse or the rare human being who does not have any sexual outlet at all, be it with another person or alone? Or is it someone who has a high sex drive but deliberately avoids any form of sexual release for whatever reason. One thing is for certain. You are not going to get this sort of information unless you are prepared to speak frankly about sex, sexuality and masturbation.

My own guiding principle is that people are entitled to privacy in their sex lives. We have no right to enquire about that part of their lives unless it can be of value in finding their homeopathic remedy. Therefore we have to ask most adults about sex and the secret of doing this well is always in your tone of voice.

Existential psychotherapy

Existential psychotherapy has much in common with the homeopathic consultation. This is due to the existential concept of bracketing, which is the existential demand on the therapist to put aside preconceived notions, attitudes and stereotypes, as these would prevent a true encounter with the uniqueness of the individual.

Let us listen to Hahnemann who wrote the following, long before the word 'existential' entered the dictionary.

> This individualising examination of a case of disease…
> demands of the physician nothing but *freedom from prejudice*
>
> *(Organon §83)*

'Freedom from prejudice'. The italics are Hahnemann's but if I had to choose one phrase from the *Organon* to shine out of this book, this would be it. It is possible to interpret the phrase in many different ways but it is greatly to Hahnemann's credit that whatever meaning you take from it, it can only make you into a better homeopath.

It could mean to be free of any of the following prejudices:

- Preconceived attitudes to people of either gender, of different race or religion, political allegiance, socio-economic status, nationality or occupation.

- Being too optimistic or pessimistic according to which orthodox diagnosis the patient presents with

- Having too early an idea of what the patient's remedy might be, for example to think of Calcarea carbonica too early in a pale-skinned, obese person thereby prejudicing you against the possibility of other remedies

- Having too strong a preference for certain types of personalities.

All this makes being 'without prejudice' a tremendously difficult task. We all have, at least, unconscious prejudices against various types of people based on our personal and social experience. I would suggest that it is almost impossible to be 'without prejudice' and perhaps the closest we can come to this is to be aware of the prejudices we do have. In the very moment of being aware of a prejudice, we disempower that particular prejudice. Also the observation of the prejudice can give us information regarding the patient as we are then using our own imperfection as a diagnostic aid.

I was strongly influenced by the particular type of existential psychotherapy developed by my first mentor in homeopathy, Dr Eric Ledermann. His medical philosophy differs from the pessimistic existentialism of Sartre and Genet. In his view the existence of a conscience in man is axiomatic, although it may appear to be absent in psychopaths. This conscience, an inherent part of a person, is not synonymous with what Freud called the 'superego', which is a collection of beliefs based on a morality set by society. According to Ledermann, most neuroses are due to this conscience existing mainly in the unconscious mind and therefore temporarily inaccessible to the patient. Patients suffer from neurotic misery because they are not in touch with their conscience as a guide on how to lead their lives. In the absence of a sincere and strong religious faith, they have little to live for and suffer in different ways in an existential vacuum. The role of an existential therapist working on this premise is simple but far from easy. It is to facilitate the process of bringing to the conscious level the unconscious conscience of the patient.

This is a profoundly optimistic view of the nature of man. Sometimes it takes the shock of a serious illness to initiate such a search within ourselves. Patients often wonder why they contracted a certain illness at any particular time. Countless patients have asked the question: 'Why did I get this now? I have been well all my life.' And yet it is obvious that any illness had to start at some time. When such a question is asked it is really an invitation to a philosophical discussion. If you, the homeopath, choose to shy away from the question by simply saying that you do not know the answers to his questions, the patient may feel that he has been rejected. There is no harm in talking about various possibilities and watching carefully how your patient handles such a conversation. Patients needing different remedies will have different views on the aetiology of their illnesses. A patient needing Phosphorus, for example, may be much more open to the idea of a psychosomatic explanation for their illness than a patient who needs Nux vomica.

The existential view of Eric Ledermann has room for the influence of: the Freudian concepts of libido, parapraxis and interpretation of dreams; the Jungian ideas of archetypes and introversion and extraversion; and even strong religious faith. However none of these are seen in a deterministic way. All are seen as challenges to be overcome by the patient, with the aid of his conscience, which is hopefully becoming more conscious as a result of the existential psychotherapy.

I find such a view to be relatively free of prejudice and a useful, ethical position to be guided by as a physician and homeopath. It is not only the patient who will suffer less if he lives according to his conscience, but the doctor as well. It is always helpful to try to put yourself in your patient's shoes and ask yourself how you would like to be treated or what you would not want said or done to you.

There was a time in history when doctors were the priests of society. The word 'doctor' actually means teacher. With the decline of institutionalised religion in the Western world and the complete separation of religion and medicine, what is left for a doctor to teach? Ledermann's approach to existentialism offers at least one piece of general advice for all patients. It is in the form of an appeal to become aware of one's conscience and then live according to it. The way in which a patient responds to this appeal will yield clues as to what homeopathic remedy might suit him best.

I am not suggesting that you insist on having discussions about ethics with every patient. It is just that I have noticed that so many patients suddenly start asking themselves questions about the meaning of life when they become ill and bring these questions to their doctors and homeopaths. I believe an honest discussion about these matters is more likely to be useful homeopathically than saying that you 'don't know' and going on to ask a standard homeopathic question. I am only suggesting that you allow the homeopathic questions to be patient-led. If the patient chooses to move into philosophical territory, you should then be able to travel with him into that arena.

It is a sad fact that most doctors do not have the inclination or the time to have such conversations with their patients. Considering philosophy of medicine unimportant, they are inadvertently adopting a philosophical position of what Ledermann has called 'naive realism'. Clearly it is unhealthy for patients and, alarmingly, even more unhealthy for doctors. Statistics consistently show that doctors are more likely than their patients to commit suicide, get divorced or become alcoholics or drug addicts. Could this be because deep down in their unconscious consciences they know they are not addressing the real reasons for which many of their patients are consulting them? If a doctor has a strong religious faith, he can be certainly be guided by that in how he treats his patients, though he must tread very carefully when there is a conflict between his faith and that of the patient over any issue. In the absence of religious faith, he could do well to look at the contribution to the philosophy of medicine and ethics of Eric Ledermann, a fine homeopath, psychiatrist and medical philosopher.

Buber

Martin Buber is worthy of our attention as it was his belief that man in a way defines himself through the quality of his relationships. In his classic text *I and Thou*[51] he differentiates between 'I-It' and 'I-Thou' relationships.

I-It relationships are those in which others are regarded as objects rather than individuals who are capable of their own, unique and subjective experience. This is more often than not the type of relationship that exists between patient and doctor in orthodox medical science.

In a short essay on Buber's influence, DeWitt and Baldwin sum this up well:

> Indeed, the scientific method is man's most highly perfected development of the I-It, or subject-object, way of knowing. It is qualified to compare object with object, even man with man, but not to know his wholeness, or his uniqueness.'[52]

This is the difference between orthodox medicine, clearly based on the scientific method, and the holistic approach of classical homeopathy, which elevates man's uniqueness to the highest possible level. In order to appreciate the ways in which a patient is unique, it is necessary for the relationship between homeopath and patient to have some of the qualities of an I-Thou relationship which is 'characterised by mutuality, directness, presentness, intensity, and ineffability'. This is what we need to strive for in our relationship with our patients. I believe that a homeopath-patient relationship with those qualities will offer up to the homeopath the information he needs to make a successful prescription.

Of course it is no simple matter to enter into such a relationship with a patient. It may take a great deal of work on yourself but it is worth considering that Buber is referring to all our relationships in his philosophy. We can only improve the quality of our relationships in the consulting room by trying to elevate all the relationships in our lives to an I-Thou level. It may be a lifetime's work but I would invite you to ask yourself whether you have something better to do with your life than to improve your relationships with your family, beloved friends, patients and fellow man in general.

I probably unconsciously chose medicine as a career because of the possibility of having such relationships with people. I was interested in the science of medicine but never fascinated by it. When forced to study and memorise mechanistic medicine in the intimidating detail demanded by medical school, I started to feel brutalised. I now know that this was because of the total focus on the I-It relationship between a medical doctor and his patient's disease. I do not want to disparage this relationship in medicine. Without it, Fleming would not have discovered penicillin and put horrendous diseases like syphilis, pneumonia and meningitis to the sword. Thousands would die or suffer unnecessarily without the sophisticated surgical techniques now at our disposal. Many treatable diseases would be undiagnosed without the magnificent investigative technology available to the modern scientific doctor. Results based on this type of medicine are based on the I-It relationship of scientific enquiry. It is, however, far from sufficient to be the only type of relationship necessary for the successful practice of medicine in general.

By far the majority of patients consulting general practitioners are coming for conditions which will not respond dramatically to the tools at the disposal of their doctor. Indeed, many studies have shown that well over half the patients consulting general practitioners are suffering from complaints that are either caused or exacerbated by psychological factors. In all these consultations the patient is going to feel that his needs have been unmet by the doctor if he is only engaged in an I-It type of relationship. Even in the most developed countries in the world, patients visiting a general practitioner are seldom allocated more than 15 minutes a visit and in the vast majority of consultations much less than that. Perhaps it is possible to have a few I-Thou moments in such a short time but the chances of this type of relationship being predominant in the average surgery must be very slim indeed. This is a sad fact for patient and doctor. Both lose the chance to experience the I-Thou relationship described by Buber. It is no less than a tragedy of modern medicine.

In the opening paragraph of this book I asked you why you wanted to be a good homeopath. When I read Buber I knew why I had been entranced by classical homeopathy. Buber, in addressing the subject of psychotherapy, had emphasised the healing effects of the I-Thou relationship above any psychological theories of human behaviour. However, classical homeopathy is able go an important step further than this and prescribe a medicine based on the fruits of an I-Thou relationship between homeopath and patient. It offers the practitioner both the possibility of experiencing the I-Thou relationship in the consulting room as well as the joy of seeing the effect on patients of correctly prescribed homeopathic remedies. This is why I think it is such a privilege to practise classical homeopathy.

In 1957 Buber entered into a famous dialogue with the American psychotherapist, Carl Rogers, with whom he had much in common. Rogers was the most important influence on the way I converse with patients and the next chapter is devoted to his view of what exactly makes a psychotherapeutic encounter (and, in my opinion, a homeopathic conversation) effective or not.

Others

Other psychologists and philosophers who have influenced me include Frankl, Maslow, Laing, Satir, Balint, Ram Das and Krishnamurti. I have tried to focus on those writers who influenced the way I saw the homeopath-patient relationship. I have no doubt that you will have been influenced and will be inspired by different groups of writers. There will always be more to learn about the homeopath-patient relationship. This, for me, is the most beautiful thing about homeopathy and probably the reason homeopaths are so unwilling to retire. When you finally start to feel comfortable and confident in the relationships you have with your patients, it must be very hard to say goodbye to the very art that encouraged those qualities in yourself – the art of the homeopathic conversation.

Chapter 9

Rogers, Counselling and Homeopathy

Towards the end of medical school I began to realise that I was not going to be taught much about communicating with patients. In my sixth and final year of study, I remember a single afternoon where we had the chance to talk to a patient on video for a few minutes and have it played back to us. The experience was a huge wake-up call for me and I will never forget it. Unfortunately that was the only chance we got to see ourselves on video in the whole six years. In fact I don't remember anybody observing me talking to a patient in all the time I was at medical school. Effective communication with patients was something you presumably taught yourself.

When as a young doctor I began studying homeopathy in 1982, talking to patients was not a major part of the course. In those days I used to take the history in the standard order described in the summary in Chapter 5. My greatest fear was that I would forget to ask the patient some important questions such as what position they slept in.

Although I had always found it easy to talk to people, I knew my communication skills could do with some polishing, so, as mentioned in Chapter 2, I enrolled for a course in counselling at what was then called the North East London Polytechnic. This turned out to be a marvellous experience. The course was very practical and the ten of us were constantly asked to practise counselling techniques on each other. We then got real feedback from our fellow students. In these exercises we had to talk about actual personal problems. You didn't have to talk about your deepest anxieties and fears but the problem you presented had to be real. Only in this way could you give genuine feedback to the student counselling you.

The course also involved some theory and the only author referred to was Carl R. Rogers. I had heard his name before, but I had no idea how influential his work had been in all forms of counselling, education and psychotherapy. It soon became obvious to me that his 'person-centred' method of talking to patients, or clients, as he preferred to call them, seemed to be totally appropriate to the homeopathic conversation. It was a total revelation to me. Finally I was being taught what I had always yearned for; how to have meaningful, helpful conversations with my patients. The course was exciting and inspiring and left me hungry to learn more.

I knew my objective to be different from my fellow students. I remember studying counselling with a policeman, two parole officers and a teacher. I was the only doctor. Most of the other students had been sponsored by their employers to attend the course in order to acquire counselling skills for specific purposes in their work. l had a slightly different agenda. I soon realised that the Rogerian counselling skills I was studying and practising would come in very useful in their own right in my career as a doctor. I had never been taught how to tell a patient that his medical investigations had confirmed a serious disease such as cancer, and, perhaps more importantly, how to respond appropriately to his reactions on hearing this. Nobody had taught me how to break the news of a patient's death to relatives and how to deal with their reactions. I felt grateful that, as a result of this course, I would be more competent as a doctor in these sorts of situations.

However, my main agenda was to improve my skill in taking homeopathic histories. I was not to be disappointed. Studying Rogerian counselling turned out to be one of the most rewarding decisions I have made so far in my ongoing pursuit to become a better homeopath.

Carl Ransom Rogers (1902–1987) became interested in psychotherapy while a student at a seminary in New York. He went on to take an MA and PhD at the Teacher's College of Columbia University. Working initially with children, he lectured at the University of Rochester and published *The Clinical Treatment of the Problem Child*[53] in 1939. In 1940, he became professor of clinical psychology at Ohio State University and published his groundbreaking work, *Counseling and Psychotherapy*,[54] in 1942. In this, and the books that followed, he introduced his particular method of therapy or counselling. The form of psychotherapy advocated by Rogers, which became commonly referred to as 'counselling', signalled a major departure from the psychotherapy of the time which was heavily influenced by psychoanalytic theory.

A major difference between the approach advocated by Rogers and analytic psychotherapy is that the Rogerian approach has no interest in analysing or interpreting unconscious processes in his clients. The therapist neither agrees nor disagrees with what the patient says. He doesn't even make the client aware of inconsistencies in what he is saying. He simply listens as the client describes his own unique experience of life and mirrors that experience back to the client. Effective 'mirroring' provides an environment in which the client is able to grow psychologically at a rate totally in his own control. Rogers described his approach as 'non-directive', 'client-centered' and 'person-centered'.

The whole point of Rogerian counselling is for the counsellor to provide the appropriate psychological environment for the client (patient) to get in touch with various feelings, desires and fears and then deal with them at his own pace. The approach has faith in the patient's innate ability to grow as a human being when in this sort of encouraging, psychological space. The job of the therapist is to provide this space in the consulting room. Effective mirroring of the psychological world of the patient is not simply a matter of technique. It is demanding on the therapist in that the conditions required for the growth and development of the client have everything to do with the psychological state of the therapist during the actual counselling sessions.

Rogers was able to simplify the whole process by describing the three vital qualities of an effective counsellor. These, in no specific order, are:

• Empathic understanding

• Unconditional positive regard

• Congruence.

As soon as I read this incredible summary of what Rogers' work is all about, I saw the common ground his counselling shared with the ideal homeopathic conversation. As homeopaths, we need to enter into, and observe, without judgement, the psychological world of our patients, in order to receive the vital mentals we need to choose a homeopathic remedy. The ideal homeopathic consultation is non-directive, client-centred and non-judgemental. As early as the sixth paragraph of the *Organon*, Hahnemann says:

> The unprejudiced observer – well aware of the futility of transcendental speculations which can receive no confirmation from experience – be his powers of penetration ever so great.
>
> *(Organon §6)*

I became aware that Rogers was saying the same thing as Hahnemann about how a homeopath (or counsellor) should conduct himself during a conversation with a patient (or client). The goals of the counsellor and the homeopath are quite different but both need to enter into the psychological world of the patient. The counsellor does this in order to provide a safe, accepting space for the client to face their problems and deal with them at his own pace. The homeopath needs to enter that very same unique, psychological world of each patient to pick up the valuable mentals on which he might be able to base a prescription. If both counsellor and homeopath are doing their jobs well, their work in the consulting room may look very much the same except for the homeopath having to take a detailed physical history as well.

If the conversations homeopaths and Rogerian counsellors have are similar and counselling is therapeutic in its own right then shouldn't the well-taken homeopathic consultation also be therapeutic? The answer is that it often is, as every homeopath knows. We are all familiar with that look of relief on a patient's face when he has trusted you enough to reveal to you the leaves, stem and root of his problem. Sometimes this is enough to have a major therapeutic effect on the patient, which is not as surprising to experienced counsellors as it is to beginner homeopaths.

At one stage in my work as a homeopath, I began to wonder if it was the consultation that was having the therapeutic effect rather than the infinitesimal doses of homeopathic medicines that were being prescribed. Eventually I designed a trial, purely for my own education. I gave all my patients their remedies in a series of numbered powders. Only one powder would be medicated, the rest being placebo. I made a note of the number of the medicated powder and made an assessment at the next consultation. If the patient's improvement began before taking the active powder, I would know that it was not a homeopathic effect. If the patient started to feel well after taking the active powder, and especially if there was an aggravation soon after that powder, I could safely give homeopathy the credit. In this way I proved, at least to my own satisfaction, that homeopathic remedies do actually work in their own right, independent of any therapeutic effect of the consultation itself.

As a homeopath, you will often be told that it is not your homeopathic remedies that help your patients. Many conventional doctors and other sceptics will ridicule the potencies we use and say that our patients get better because of the quality and length of time of our consultations. I used to argue the point with them but it got boring after a few such conversations. I now use a different strategy. If an orthodox medical colleague tells me I am getting my patients better by the quality of my consultations, I thank him for the compliment. I then ask him why he doesn't cure his patients by talking to them as that is surely preferable to the prescription of a drug. The answer is invariably the same. ' I don't have the time' to which I remark in a sympathetic, slightly ironic voice: 'What a pity that you don't have the time to heal your patients just by listening and talking to them.' That tends to end the conversation and it is generally much more enjoyable than repetitive arguments about placebos, potencies, succussion and dilutions!

So, having made it clear that I am convinced of the clinical effectiveness of the homeopathic remedies themselves, let us return to the consultation itself. I have compared entering into someone's psychological world to watching a movie of their life. As I listen to the story of my patient's life, images come to me in much the same way as a biographical movie. The images are not as clear as film and I do not know whether these images come from my own imagination or I am picking something up from the psyche of the patient or a combination of both. What I do know is that the clarity of these images as well as the intuitive feeling that I am hearing the true story of my patient's 'dis-ease', is dependent on one thing. And that 'thing' is my own state of mind during the homeopathic conversation. I am now sure that this is by far the most important single factor that will determine how successful I am on any given working day in my consulting room. I know that if I study the materia medica for five hours a day for the rest of my life, I will not improve my homeopathic results as much as doing an hour's work on myself a day. It is my experience that being fully 'present' for my patient during the consultation is the most important factor in the making of a successful homeopathic prescription.

As this became more and more true for me and my practice, I felt compelled to change the way I studied homeopathy. Of course I continued to sit in on the consultations of more experienced homeopaths, but I also began to look at what the various psychotherapy schools had to say about the therapist-client relationship. My goal was to take what was useful in the context of the homeopathic consultation and leave the rest.

Rogerian counselling was by far my biggest influence. Rogers' view was that results in psychotherapy had little to do with the intellectual prowess or knowledge of psychological theory of the counsellor. Good results were much more dependent on the counsellor's ability to own the three psychological qualities necessary to provide the right atmosphere for his client to make progress. It is this very same atmosphere that we classical homeopaths need to provide for our patients, so they can feel safe enough to tell us the true story of their illness and life.

It is worth looking at these three qualities and asking yourself how highly you rate yourself in each. By doing this you will able to see what work you need to do on yourself to improve your case-taking skills and become a better homeopath.

Empathic understanding

It is not enough for your patient to know that you feel sympathetic towards them. Those of you who have young children will know that a child is capable of feeling sympathy for you when you feel sad or anxious. This sympathy may be of some comfort but it lacks understanding of why you are 'feeling down'. Empathy is the ability to identify yourself with the patient in your consulting room; to put yourself in their shoes and get some inkling of how they are feeling. Empathic understanding means that you both intellectually understand the plight of the patient and are able to identify with how he is feeling 'in the moment'.

Even this is not enough. The patient has to be made aware of your empathic understanding. Most of the time this will happen at a non-verbal level but there are times when you may have to say something to show that you both understand and feel what he is going through. Non-interpretative comments can be helpful such as:

• 'That must have been a difficult time for you'

• 'You must have been very upset by that'

• 'That must have been painful...'

Notice that all these comments are neutral, neither commending nor condemning in the least way. It may be obvious not to condemn, but if you praise one statement and don't praise the next one, the withholding of praise may be experienced by the patient as criticism. This is a difficult lesson to learn as we all want to say things that make our patients feel better.

In identifying with the patient's feelings, it is vital not to lose a sense of yourself. This means remaining aware of a psychological boundary between your patient's life and your own. If you become overwhelmed by the patient's feelings you will not be able to provide a safe environment for him to express more feelings and in this way you may miss out on hearing vital homeopathic clues. In an emotionally charged situation this can feel like walking a tightrope with no safety-net in sight. Saying the wrong thing can be disastrous, and remaining silent may give the patient the impression that you don't care.

However, we can never hope to remain in a state of empathic understanding for all of the time in every consultation. I have found that it is almost impossible to *try* to be empathic. Either you are empathic or understanding in the moment or you are not. So what can be done to improve this quality in yourself? My only suggestion is to observe yourself very carefully when you see your own lack of empathy, for any reason, when you are consulting. Do not chastise yourself in any way and don't feel guilty. Simply observe the truth of the moment. In the very moment that you acknowledge and feel your own lack of empathy, there is the possibility there and then of regaining empathic understanding.

Unconditional positive regard

This means that the therapist should adopt a kind or even loving attitude to his client no matter who the client is or what he says. In suggesting this as an attribute of an effective counsellor, Rogers appears to be implying that he believes that all people have a positive nature at the deepest possible level. Therefore no matter what the therapist sees on the surface, he should strive to have positive regard for the goodness within all his clients. He is therefore not entitled to judge his client in any way. This is a clear philosophical position and a very optimistic assessment of the human condition. If all men are worthy of unconditional positive regard, then there must be goodness in the hearts of us all. As Rogers puts it: 'I have always been able to rely on the fact that if I can get through the shell, if I can get through to the person, there will be a positive and constructive inner core.' [55]

I feel Rogers' view here to be consistent with that of my teacher, Eric Ledermann, who believes that the great majority of human beings have a conscience. Neurotic misery will end if we are able to make that conscience conscious and live according to it. It is therefore possible to have unconditional positive regard for the conscience of every patient and believe in their capacity to get in touch with that conscience at their own pace and to live by it. (The exception to the rule is in the case of the psychopath or sociopath where there appears to be an absence of a conscience and no remorse for causing pain to others.)

I have sometimes seen Rogers' 'unconditional positive regard' referred to as 'warmth' which is something with which I feel more comfortable. Warmth conveys to me a sense of a friendly acceptance of whatever the patient may be feeling at any time during the conversation, be it dismay, anger, resentment, anxiety, fear, pride or joy. All emotions are warmly accepted as parts of the whole and it is the whole individual that is valued by the 'person-centred approach'.

This non-judgemental acceptance is of great relevance to the classical homeopath and is entirely consistent with Hahnemann's phrase, 'freedom from prejudice'. If a patient thinks that any aspect of his personality will be judged or criticised, even silently, by his homeopath, he will not reveal that side of himself. It is exactly the information that the patient would hide from you if he feels judged, that you need when it comes to analysing the case. Why should he make himself vulnerable if there is a chance of being judged unfavourably? But if he feels his whole being to be warmly and unconditionally accepted in the moment, he will be more likely to take a chance and tell you the true story of himself.

How do you develop 'unconditional positive regard' or warmth towards your patients? Like empathy, it is not something that can be attained by an act of will. I think it is almost impossible to have unconditional positive regard for every patient who steps into your consulting room. There will always be people we simply cannot bring ourselves to like. This is due to our complex nature as human beings. When I find myself judging a patient or unable to feel warmly towards him, I try to ask myself why this is so. The most frequent answer I get to this question is that up to the point of asking the question, I have unconsciously noticed in my patient a feature in myself that I dislike or am unable to accept. I then try to admit this to myself and accept myself as a whole in the moment. If I can accept the imperfection in myself, I can simultaneously accept it in my patient. The homeopathic consultation becomes an opportunity for growth for the homeopath himself. It is not every profession that offers such rewards.

I have been asked: 'What happens when you believe you just cannot feel "positive regard" for your patient?' This is possible, but is quite a rare occurrence in my experience. If you cannot feel the necessary warmth towards a patient, you should probably refer them to another homeopath and explain to that homeopath why you needed to do this. The discussion you have with him will help him a lot in understanding his new patient as well as help him choose a remedy.

It is essential to remember why you first wanted to become a homeopath. In most cases a love of humanity is at least on the list. As time goes by we can be tempted to 'be practical' and focus on the business side of things, but while the spark of love that took you into homeopathy can appear dim at times, it never goes out. If you can dispassionately observe that dimming, you may suddenly feel it burst into flame inside you.

Congruence

This quality, which has also been described by Rogers as 'genuineness', 'realness' and 'authenticity', is essential if you want to become a competent homeopath. In my opinion it is an absolute requirement for a homeopath to be as genuine as possible at all times in the consultation. The alternative is to hide behind the mask of a 'professional' facade. The worst possible thing you can do in a homeopathic conversation is to wear any sort of mask, thereby hiding your real self from your patient. There is nothing more disconcerting for a patient than the feeling that his doctor or homeopath lacks authenticity at any time during the consultation. If he senses that you are not being genuine at any moment, the consultation will be ruined.

Would you confide in someone who you sensed was putting on an act, or hiding behind a cheerful mask, or not being genuine in the moment? I know that I would not. If you cannot trust yourself enough to be yourself in the moment, then why should your patients trust you with the most intimate details of their lives? If you are confident enough to be yourself, imperfect as you are, in the consultation room, then your patient will find himself in an atmosphere in which he too will feel comfortable about expressing himself genuinely. If you don't wear a mask yourself your patients will be encouraged to drop theirs and trust you with the truth.

The need to be genuine in the homeopathic conversation may seem obvious but the sad truth is that much human interaction takes place between people wearing masks. You will not need to look too far to see a fake smile or an inauthentic look of concern. People are scared of showing their real feelings to the world, sometimes for very good reasons. There are those who would exploit the weaknesses of others and so people wear masks for self-preservation. That is why they need to feel safe enough in your consulting room to be themselves. Empathy and warmth can be extremely useful in this regard, but authenticity in the homeopath is essential.

I am not suggesting that you articulate every feeling you have while talking to your patients. In an interview published in the year of his death, Rogers said:

> When I am with a client, I like to be aware of my feelings, and if there are feelings which run contrary to the conditions of therapy and occur persistently, then I am sure I want to express them. But there are also other feelings. For instance, sometimes, with a woman client, I feel: 'this woman is sexually attractive, I feel attracted to her.' I would not express that unless it comes up as an issue in therapy. But, if I felt annoyed that she was always complaining, let us say, and I kept feeling annoyed, then, I would express it. The important thing is to be aware of one's feeling and then you can decide whether it needs to be expressed or is appropriate to express.[56]

This is authenticity. You don't have to express all that you feel. It is possible to be genuine in silence as well. It is simply a matter of being yourself. In an inspirational footnote to paragraph 141 of the *Organon*, Hahnemann writes:

> Again, by such noteworthy observations on himself he will be brought to understand his own sensations, his mode of thinking and his disposition (the foundation of all true wisdom, γνωθι σεαυτ῀Ον ('know yourself'), and he will be also trained to be, what every physician ought to be, a good observer.
>
> *(Organon §141)*

Paragraph 141 is actually about the homeopath proving medicines on himself. To understand the changes a medicine produces in you, it is important to 'know yourself' before taking it. However when Hahnemann uses a phrase like 'the foundation of all true wisdom' in relation to knowing yourself it is clear he is applying the necessity to 'know yourself' to a much wider context than the provings.

For me 'know yourself' is one of those phrases from the Organon like 'without prejudice' that hint at the awesome responsibility involved in becoming a good homeopath. When exactly can anyone say 'I now know myself' or 'I am now without prejudice'? Any homeopath saying this would be as unlikely to be believed as one saying: 'I now know the homeopathic materia medica.' What is being suggested by both Hahnemann and Rogers is not an endpoint but a journey. A journey of self-discovery on which every homeopath should be embarking. How else can we know ourselves, as well as having the courage to be true to ourselves at all times, especially in the consulting room? Is it possible to be true to ourselves only while consulting? I think not. The only mask that does not exist is the mask of authenticity. Authenticity is the face behind all the other masks most of us wear at different times.

There are no easy paths to authenticity, self-knowledge or love. This is why Rogerian counselling is simple but very demanding. The knowledge you have to acquire is self-knowledge – which Hahnemann described as 'the foundation of all true wisdom'. The main thing is to realise that a journey to self-knowledge is a necessity. In what vehicle you choose to travel is entirely up to you.

James Tyler Kent and many of his followers were Swedenborgians. This was the vehicle they used for their own spiritual journeys. Kent does not advocate the study of Swedenborgianism for homeopaths but he has made clear that he saw a strong resonance between what was said by Hahnemann and Swedenborg.

Kent and many of his colleagues were clearly on a spiritual journey and their practice of homeopathy was completely compatible with their religious or spiritual beliefs. The spiritual path they were on probably inspired them to produce some of the finest homeopathic books ever written. Kent's *Repertory*[57] and *Lectures on Materia Medica*[58] are obvious examples, but the works of Boericke, Hempel, Guernsey and Farrington, all Swedenborgians, remain classics of homeopathic literature.

I have always been interested in the religions, spiritual paths, or 'growth work' that have inspired or continue to inspire other homeopaths. Some are willing to talk openly about this aspect of their lives while others are much more private about it. I have never been afraid to ask my colleagues if they practise a religion or follow a spiritual path. Sometimes this has led to honest, authentic conversations that have been an inspiration for me. Others have been more private about this aspect of their lives, as is their right.

In nearly two decades of practising homeopathy and attending many courses and seminars, I have met many classical homeopaths from all over the world. It is has become clear to me that many of them are involved in some inner journey or spiritual path. These have included: all the major Western and Eastern institutionalised religions (with special emphasis on the spiritual dimension); yoga; t'ai chi and most of the other martial arts; Zen; psychoanalysis and all the different types of psychotherapy; and many different groups following charismatic leaders or gurus. I have yet to meet a classical homeopath who declared himself to be an atheist.

Codes of ethics, religions, spiritual groups and even the different psychoanalytic groups may have different names, holy books, teachers and leaders. This is less important than simply asking yourself whether the path you are on is working for you. The destination is less important than the intuitive feeling that you are making progress in the right direction.

At the end of medical school, at the age of 24, I was obliged to take the Hippocratic Oath (reproduced in full in the appendix at the end of this book). It meant a lot to me then, and still does now. It has fallen out of favour to the extent that very few medical schools include it even as an option for their students. Perhaps they consider some of Hippocrates' admonitions to be outmoded or too severe for comfort. That is a matter of conjecture but one thing that can be said of the oath is that it gives deep consideration to the mental and spiritual health of the physician. Hippocrates was clearly concerned that physicians looked after themselves psychologically and spiritually. As was mentioned in Chapter 8, doctors are less likely to be looking after themselves than are the public at large. In my opinion, the orthodox medical profession as a whole is suffering from an epidemic of 'burnout'.

This is less true of homeopaths, and that is one of the reasons why it is a privilege and a pleasure to be teaching classical homeopathy to doctors. Some doctors have been 'cured' of burnout by their studying and practising of homeopathy. However, we classical homeopaths are by no means immune from burning out and I have seen it happen to talented colleagues.

When I first heard the expression 'physician heal thyself', I used to feel inadequate as a doctor. This is because I interpreted it as implying that doctors should heal themselves first before attempting to help others. Now I feel that what this means is that physicians should be in the process of healing themselves. This, for me, is the same journey to authenticity recommended by Hahnemann in the footnote to paragraph 143. It is what Rogers means by congruence, genuineness and authenticity. To have these qualities permanently locked into us may seem impossible. Nevertheless we can try to remain on the path towards them. And when we inevitably slip off the path, we should not be too self-critical as we struggle to continue on the journey. Why should we, homeopaths and wounded healers ourselves, not be as gentle with ourselves as we are with our patients?

When I feel I need inspiration as a doctor and homeopath, I often think of the following three little pieces of advice from three gifted clinicians. They shouldn't be too hard to remember as they comprise exactly seven words in total!

Physician heal thyself (Biblical)

Know yourself (Hahnemann)

Be yourself (Rogers)

Carl Rogers is best known for advocating the qualities of congruence, empathic understanding and unconditional positive regard for therapists and counsellors. In doing this, he departed from the analytically influenced, psychotherapeutic theory of his time. Together with Maslow and others he helped usher in the era of humanistic psychology. This differs from psychoanalytic theory in that instead of seeing human behaviour as the product of unconscious forces and conditioning, it believes that people have free will and the ability to change if given an appropriate psychological environment. Humanistic psychology is optimistic in its belief that human beings have the capacity to grow and change for the better if they feel understood and loved by therapists who are authentic in themselves.

The humanistic approach claims to be able to effect change in far fewer sessions than the analytic approach which may require several sessions a week for many years. Humanistic psychotherapy has thus been able to make itself available to a far greater number of people and has had a profound influence on many professionals in the fields of medicine, education and even crisis telephone helplines.

Towards the end his life, Rogers said: 'it does not make much fundamental difference whether the client sees me as a young person or a lover, or as a father figure, as long as the client is able to express some of those feelings. The process is the same regardless of which feelings are being expressed.'

For us as homeopaths, the expression of these feelings by our patients is also crucial, but exactly which feelings are expressed, will have a huge influence on our choice of a homeopathic remedy.

I have referred to the psychological process called transference, about which Rogers goes on to say the following:

This is why I differ so fundamentally with the psychoanalysts on this business of transference. I think it is quite natural that a client might feel positive feelings towards the therapist. There is no reason to make a big deal out of it. It can be handled in the same way as the fact that the client might be afraid of the therapist, or of his or her father. Any feelings are grist for the mill as far as therapy is concerned, providing the client can express them and providing the therapist is able to listen acceptantly. I think the whole concept of transference got started because the therapist got scared when the client began to feel strong positive or negative feelings towards the therapist. The whole process of therapy is a process of self-exploration, of getting aquainted with one's own feelings and coming to accept them as a part of the self. So, whether the feelings are in regard to the parents, or in regard to the therapist, or in regard to some situation, it really makes no difference. The client is better aquainted with and becoming more accepting of his or her self and that can be true with regard to the transference feelings. When the client realises: 'Yes, I do love him very much,' or whatever and accepts those as a real part of self, the process of therapy advances.[59]

I find this insightful, inspiring and entirely appropriate advice for classical homeopaths. I strongly recommend that you read the passage above again, this time substituting the words 'therapist' and 'client' with 'homeopath' and 'patient'. Any feelings expressed by our patients, for whatever reason, are not only 'grist for the mill' as far as therapy is concerned, they are the very stuff on which many a successful homeopathic prescription is made.

Over the course of his career Rogers expressed many other ideas, some of which are very useful to homeopaths. Others, such as his pioneering work with encounter groups and his views on education, are less relevant to us, and will not be discussed. However his belief in the recording of live case histories is extremely relevant to homeopathic education.

Tape recording of case histories

Carl Rogers was the first psychotherapist to record cases of psychotherapy. Even before the age of the tape recorder, he was recording his sessions with patients on early, metallic recording devices, showing tremendous courage and confidence in what he was doing and a willingness to share his knowledge and skills with his students in the most effective way possible.

He went on to embrace the tape recorder and the video recorder as well as doing therapy in front of live audiences. I have been personally 'therapped' in front of both a video camera and a live audience at the same time and not felt the slightest impediment to the therapeutic process. If anything, it intensified the therapeutic process. In my case, I felt empathy and even admiration from the audience, for having the courage to do this.

Many classical homeopaths are now recording case histories on videotape. In the majority of cases the video camera is pointed only at the patient. This is for teaching purposes so that homeopathic students can see, for example, a Calcarea phosphorica patient before and after the administration of the remedy. This is invaluable in teaching materia medica and case analysis. I feel it can also be of great use in teaching case-taking skills simply by pointing the video camera at the homeopath for the duration of the consultation. We will discuss this further in Chapter 18.

Chapter 10

Techniques in the Consulting Room

In the previous chapter, we focused on the qualities that a good counsellor or homeopath needs to develop in himself in order to become more proficient in taking the case. There is nothing more important than the gradual process of recognising and accepting one's own imperfections in order to be able to accept our patients' imperfections (or symptoms) in authentic conversation.

Unfortunately this process may well take the better part of a lifetime, so we also need to find other methods of improving the quality of our case-taking. In this chapter I will share with you the various ways I have been able to improve my case-taking skills over the last 20 years as well as my ongoing explorations in my favourite part of the homeopathic process – talking to patients. The list of techniques and influences explored here is by no means comprehensive. It is important for me to confine the discussion to what has worked for me, personally. If I were to write hypothetically about techniques that look good on paper, but are untried in my own practice, I would be joining the ranks of those homeopaths who have written materia medicae based on what others have said about the remedies, rather than on what they have observed in their own clinical experience.

Neurolinguistic programming (NLP)

Neurolinguistic programming, commonly known as NLP, is a method of influencing human behaviour by the employment of specific observational skills and psychological techniques of proven efficacy.

Initially developed by Richard Bandler and John Grinder, it is now taught in seminars in institutes all over the world. It has applications in medicine, psychology, education, industry and sales techniques. It is also used one to one in a similar format to psychotherapy or more specifically, hypnotherapy. I attended a few seminars to see if NLP could help improve the way I was taking the case in homeopathy. My aim was not to qualify as a neurolinguistic programmer. I wanted to take from it what might be useful in homeopathic consulting, try those techniques out for myself and ignore the rest. Interestingly, this is similar to the way NLP itself developed.

Bandler and Grinder developed NLP by observing famous psychotherapists who were reputed to be getting excellent clinical results. Three therapists were major influences: the hypnotherapist Milton Erickson; the family therapist Virginia Satir; and the founder of Gestalt, Fritz Perls.

Their view was that effective psychotherapists were certainly getting results but not for the reasons they thought they were. Rogers was saying something similar in that he thought any form of therapy could be effective if the therapist had the internal qualities of empathy, warmth and congruence. Grinder and Bandler, however, focused on the external, visible methods and behaviour of the people they studied. From these observations they collated what they perceived to be effective in the consultations they observed, and called it NLP. This was the start and NLP has developed since then with a growing literature on the subject, in all its various applications. A summary of these would be long and pointless in the context of this book. I will just share with you a few ideas I have picked up from NLP and that have been helpful in the consulting room.

NLP recognises that rapport between patient and therapist is vital for good results in psychotherapy. They noticed that effective therapists seemed to be unconsciously matching the physical movements and even breathing of their patients. Thus they 'modelled' this process. You could consciously match your breathing to your patient's breathing, apparently helping increase the rapport between you. To me this felt much too contrived, as did much of NLP. There is a difference between unconscious matching of behaviour which is based on genuine rapport and a conscious, premeditated attempt to create rapport by copying the patient's behaviour. I did not feel comfortable with it and do not use it. That is not to say that it may not be effective. It just failed the 'authenticity test' for me.

A very important contribution of NLP is its observation of how different people use their senses in different ways. We all pick up information with our eyes (visual), our ears (auditory) and touch (kinaesthetic). NLP has shown that we all favour one of these above the other two in the way we relate to the external world. One of the three tends to be dominant. I know, for example, that I am more auditory than visually articulate. I cannot remember what colour dress someone was wearing or notice road signs from afar, but I have little problem remembering the words of poems or the lyrics of songs. My wife, an artist and art therapist, has incredible visual acuity and remembers the visual details from films, as well as having excellent recall of her clients' art images. I am pretty sure that this is not a gender differentiation, though I once saw a greeting card with the joke: Behind every successful woman is a man (turn the card) asking 'Where are my socks?'.

Other people may be more kinaesthetically dominant. I remember someone telling me the following hypothetical conversation between a visually dominant husband and a kinaesthetically dominant wife to show how rapport can be lost when both partners are unaware that they have different dominant senses.

Husband: *(coming home to an untidy house) The house is in a terrible mess. How can you live in this? Can't you see the chaos around you?*

This is unlikely to effect any change in behaviour on the part of his wife. The truth is that being a kinaesthetically dominant person, she really does not see the mess around her.

Now, supposing the husband, having studied a little NLP, knew that he was visually dominant and his wife was kinaesthetically dominant. He might then have addressed her in the following way.

Husband: *When I see the house in a mess like this I feel as annoyed as you do when I eat toast in bed and spill crumbs.*

Wife: *Oh, lord, I hate that, the crumbs… yes, okay, I'll try to keep the house a bit more tidy, but don't eat toast in bed ever again.*

The second approach was more effective because the wife responded to words and images appropriate for someone whose kinaesthetic sense was dominant.

Patients may tell you which sense is dominant by the words they use as shown below.

• Kinaesthetically dominant people
  I feel
  I feel down
  I have a gut feeling
  That makes me feel…

- Visually dominant people
  I see
  I see what you mean
  I get the picture

- Auditory dominant people
  I hear you
  It sounds like

NLP trains you to recognise words used by the patient that help you locate their dominant sense. You can then use words in the same paradigm to communicate with your patient rather than words appropriate to your own dominant sense. Apparently this works very well in making good contact with patients, and there are homeopaths who have trained in NLP. I found the whole process too contrived and manipulative to feel comfortable using it. However, I also found that when I had managed to establish rapport with a patient, I seemed to be practising some of the NLP 'techniques' without realising it.

Nevertheless, I do believe that homeopaths can learn case-taking skills from NLP. Perhaps it needs a classical homeopath who has also been fully trained in NLP, to teach us what exactly in NLP is appropriate and useful in the homeopathic consultation.

Humour

A sense of humour is a tremendously useful tool in the homeopathic conversation – just as it is in any social conversation. When a patient genuinely laughs with his homeopath, this often confirms that rapport has been established. It has to be genuine laughter, of course. Fake smiles and forced laughter do not indicate rapport at all. They are sad things to witness in any conversation and should always be regarded as symptoms in the homeopathic context.

The use of humour in medicine and homeopathy should never be contrived. Still, we do hear a lot of very funny things from our patients and they too are often aware of the funny side of what they are saying. If a patient says something that really amuses me I allow myself to laugh openly. As I am amused by a lot of things in life, I often find myself laughing during homeopathic conversations. In most cases I find that my patient is laughing with me. We both relax and the conversation moves into a higher gear. I have laughed with patients who were suffering from very severe disease and have felt quite comfortable doing so. In such cases I have felt that we have been laughing at life itself and the predicaments it throws at us.

I seldom feel guilty about laughing while I am consulting. I feel that if I held back the laughter, I would be inauthentic in the moment and that would be an obstacle to rapport. I never laugh *at* patients. It is just that the predicaments they find themselves in, sometimes entirely of their own making, are sometimes very amusing – and they know it.

Of course there have been a few times when I have laughed inappropriately. This is no different from inadvertently saying something that upsets the patient. We have all experienced this and know what it feels like. The way to repair the damage is always the same – a genuine apology, full of warmth and empathic understanding.

Patients, who come into my consulting room with a plastic bag full of the latest vitamins, minerals and other food supplements for me to analyse usually get the following piece of advice: 'Remember it is not only what you eat that is important, it is also what is eating you!' Whether the patient likes this humorous little truism or not, it often pushes the subject of conversation away from nutrition and towards emotion.

In addition to helping create rapport, laughter has been scientifically proven to: improve our breathing; increase our immunity to infection; reduce our levels of adrenaline and nor-adrenaline (the hormones of fight and flight); reduce muscular tension; as well as being an excellent form of exercise. And that list does not even included the obvious psychological and spiritual benefits of laughter.

There is a lot of truth in the cliché, 'many a true word is said in jest'. Sometimes the truth is so painful for people that the most compassionate way of communicating it is in jest. This has always been the role of the court jester. One of the best examples of this in literature is in Shakespeare's masterpiece, *King Lear*. In the play, Lear, in old age, decides to give away his kingdom to his three daughters. His two older daughters flatter him to obtain their inheritance but the youngest refuses to boost his ego by doing this. He gradually loses all his power and even the love of the two daughters who, after accepting their inheritance, grow tired of having their ageing father around.

His ego receives a succession of painful blows until he is left without a home, defenceless against a raging storm. With the destruction of his ego and power comes an element of self-knowledge, but that is all Shakespeare allows him, as the play ends in tragedy with the death of Cordelia, the daughter who had rejected her inheritance, but maintained her love for her father. As Lear agonisingly loses his power, and nearly his mind, he is mercilessly teased by his court jester, or 'fool', who takes every chance available to hold up a comic mirror to the truth of his master's painful decline. Lear's fool coaxes him with humour towards honesty and self-knowledge.

> *Fool:* Dost thou know the difference, my boy, between a bitter fool and a sweet one?
>
> *Lear:* No lad, teach me.
>
> *Fool:* That lord that counselled thee
> To give away thy land,
> Come place him here by me –
> Do thou for him stand.
>
> The sweet and bitter fool
> Will presently appear;
> The one in motley here,
> The other found out there.
>
> *Lear:* Dost thou call me fool, boy?
>
> *Fool:* All thy other titles thou hast given away; that thou wast born with.
>
> *Kent:* This is not altogether fool, my lord.
>
> *(Act I Scene iv)*[60]

In the homeopathic context such humour would be far too cruel, but a comforting joke can put a patient at ease and may lead to him saying something he might otherwise have chosen to withhold.

Provocation

My own case of the man who was furious for my lack of punctuality is a good example of how a patient can sometimes be provoked into acting out homeopathic information in front of one's eyes. The vision of his seething fury was so powerful that I can still see it now. This is quite different from a patient telling you that he can be 'angry at times'.

I cannot advocate the deliberate provocation of patients in this way though I have seen homeopaths do this quite successfully. One of my colleagues described the following little chat with a female patient.

Homeopath: *Do you ever feel jealous?*

Patient: *No, not really.*

Homeopath: *So if you came home early one day and caught your husband in bed with another woman, you wouldn't really mind?*

Patient: *(shocked) Well that is different. I would…*

Now this homeopath might use that ridiculous little scenario whenever he thinks he can get away with it. After using it a few times he will notice there are a variety of emotional responses to his provocative remark. The way in which any patient responds to the provocation will say something about their constitution and of course, their constitutional remedy. This is an example of deliberate provocation and is perhaps suitable only for the more mischievous homeopath.

It is possible and indeed probable that you will occasionally provoke a patient inadvertently. Before you apologise be sure to register their emotional response to your unintentionally provocative remark. It's all grist for the mill when it comes to analysing the case.

A few years ago, I met a wonderful psychotherapist by the name of Frank Farrelly. After practising Rogerian client-centred therapy for a few decades he found that although he was getting reasonable results, he felt he could be doing a lot better. He found the reflective nature of client-centred therapy a little tame to produce results quickly. In his experience, patients with low self-esteem (the most common 'mental' of all in my experience) felt better during the therapy sessions but began to deflate as soon as they left.

He wondered what would happen if instead of trying in any way to raise their self-esteem, he simply agreed with what they said about themselves and even exaggerated it a little. He immediately discovered that when patients with low self-esteem ('doormats' as he calls them) heard him agreeing with their critical assessment of themselves, these 'doormats stood up on their hind legs and started to defend themselves'. This led him to explore other ways of provoking self-affirmative responses, such as offering idiotic solutions to the patients' problems; pointing out advantages to their problems; mimicking them; wandering off on irrational tangents to the topic and interrupting them. Eventually he called his brand of psychotherapy 'Provocative Therapy' and wrote a wonderful book with that title.[61]

The most important thing about Provocative Therapy is that it must be done with an open heart. Empathic understanding and unconditional positive regard are vital. If you provoke a patient without using warmth, it will feel as though you are being sadistic. But if 'with a twinkle in your eye and affection in your heart' (in Farrelly's words), you gently satirise the patient's self-limiting beliefs about himself, you may be surprised by how he responds.

Frank Farrelly told me that a homeopathic physician attending one of his seminars once compared Provocative Therapy to homeopathy. He claimed that what Farrelly was doing was taking the symptoms of the patient, diluting (potentising) them with humour and giving them back to the patient. Obviously this is not the same as giving a potentised homeopathic remedy but I found the comparison interesting.

This is how Farrelly describes the goals of Provocative Therapy.

The provocative therapist attempts to create both positive and negative affective experiences in an effort to provoke the client to engage in five different types of behaviour:

1. To affirm his self-worth, both verbally and behaviourally.

2. To assert himself appropriately both in task performances and relationships.

3. To defend himself realistically.

4. To engage in psycho-social reality testing and learn the necessary discriminations to respond adaptively. Global perceptions lead to global stereotyped responses; differentiated perceptions lead to adaptive responses.

5. To engage in risk-taking behaviours in personal relationships, especially communicating affection and vulnerability to significant others with immediacy as they are authentically experienced by the client. The most difficult words in relationships are often 'I want you, I miss you, I care about you' – to commit oneself to others.

Provocation in the homeopathic consultation is bound to sound like sacrilege to some homeopaths, especially those who feel that a homeopath should sit quietly and wait for the symptoms. However, even sitting quietly can be provocative as in the previously mentioned case of Dr Somper's patient who, growing increasingly impatient with his silence, burst out with: 'Don't just sit there, do something!' – leading to a successful prescription of Chamomilla.

For homeopaths who enjoy a laugh, are prepared to take a chance when the situation feels right and enjoy the odd tease, the occasional provocative remark can prove to be a surprisingly effective way of acquiring useful homeopathic information.

Words

It is essential for homeopaths to understand that words are only words and what a patient says is only a description of what he is actually feeling and who he really is. Different words mean different things to different people. People who are envious of others may incorrectly describe themselves as 'jealous'. I understand envy to be a feeling of uneasiness or even ill-will towards another person because they have an attribute or possession you desire but do not own. Jealousy, however, I understand to be an overprotection of what one feels is one's own, particularly in regard to close relationships. Those are my understandings of those two words but yours may be slightly different. The point here is that you need to know what your patient is feeling and expressing in the words he chooses.

Talking about your own life

Since leaving medical school, the most important lesson that I have learned about consulting is not to rely exclusively on my medical and homeopathic education. I now know that I am much more effective as a homeopath if I allow myself to be influenced by knowledge gained from anything, anyone and anywhere. I realise that the most direct and reliable knowledge I have of life is from my own experience of life itself.

If what a patient is saying to me resonates with a memorable experience from my own life story, I will sometimes choose to share that memory with my patient. I do not use this technique frequently but it has on occasion proven to be effective at creating rapport. Being honest about one's own life can encourage a patient to be honest and open about his own.

I remember a young female patient telling me about a problem with her boyfriend. I told her that I would have been happy to have had such a problem when I was her age because at that time in my life girls were not interested in me at all. As I said this, she smiled, visibly relaxed and even offered a few words of sympathy for me! This was the turning point in the consultation. From then on she trusted me enough to give me an honest appraisal of herself instead of complaining about her boyfriend's behaviour. Freudians would not approve of this overt expression of what they would surely label as 'counter-transference' but our goal as homeopaths is to get the information we need to prescribe accurately. Being honest about my own life provided the appropriate psychological environment for her to be honest about herself.

You may choose never to talk about your own life in the consulting room. If it feels uncomfortable for you to do so, then it is best that you do not. I think a homeopath should only ever say what feels natural, comfortable and safe in the moment. Anything contrived will sound phoney and make your patient feel uncomfortable. Being true to yourself is sometimes the key that opens the door for your patient to do the same.

There are obviously many more strategies and techniques to be deployed in the consultation. This is what makes taking the history such a fascinating part of homeopathy. Homeopaths come from different cultures and backgrounds and will have had different experiences of life.

A homeopath who is married and has children will relate differently to families from one who is single. I don't think I fully appreciated what parents meant by 'sleep deprivation' until my son was born – a good 15 years after I started practising homeopathy. This is the simple difference between sympathy and empathy. The intellectual understanding rarely matches the understanding as a result of experience. If you have suffered a bereavement yourself or been through any traumatic experience, such as a divorce, it will be easier for you to have empathy for someone who is going through a similar experience. In this way, all your life experiences, pleasurable or painful, can help you in your discussions with patients. As we, classical homeopaths, grow older (and hopefully wiser with our own experience of life) empathic understanding becomes more spontaneous. Time makes better homeopaths of us all.

Chapter 11

Time

How much time do you have for your patients ? How much of that time consists of high quality homeopathic conversation?

The amount of time allocated by homeopaths for their consultations varies enormously. I know many homeopaths who spend as long as two-and-a-half hours on the first consultation and have heard of one who may spend as long as four hours on the initial visit. These homeopaths tend to allocate between half an hour and an hour for follow-up visits. This sort of homeopath is unlikely to see more than ten patients a day. In the Western world it is possible to earn a reasonable living this way. However in India, the country that has easily the most homeopathic practitioners in the world, this is simply not possible. It is not uncommon for a homeopath in India to see close to 100 patients a day. So the actual time spent with a patient may be as long as four hours or as short as two or three minutes. Of course, homeopaths who are pressed for time may consider it an unimaginable luxury to talk to a patient for a couple of hours. On the other hand, the homeopaths working more slowly may think it 'impossible' to see 100 patients a day.

On this issue, I will defer not to Hahnemann but to Einstein. It really is all relative. It is not the amount of time spent that makes a difference – it is what *happens* in that time that is the essence of the homeopathic conversation.

In this famous opening stanza of his 'Auguries of Innocence', William Blake (1757–1827), writing just before Hahnemann but at least a century before Einstein, shows an intuitive understanding of relativity.

> To see a World in a Grain of a Sand
> And Heaven in a Wild Flower.
> Hold Infinity in the palm of your hand
> And Eternity in an hour.[62]

The first two lines can also be read as an exquisitely succinct expression of the homeopathic concepts of the infinitesimal dose and the invisible power inherent in minerals and flowers.

One wonders what Blake would have thought of the *Organon*. I was fascinated to discover that the famous English homeopath, John Henry Clarke, had written several books on Blake's work. One cannot help but wonder where the prolific author of classic homeopathic texts such as the monumental *Dictionary of Practical Materia Medica*,[63] *The Prescriber*[64] and many others, found the time to write books on poetry appreciation! Perhaps people were inclined to be more creative in the days before television insinuated itself into most of our lives.

In the context of the homeopathic conversation, the length of the consultation is less important than the quality of time spent with your patient. 'Quality time' between homeopath and patient refers to the time in consultation where there is good rapport.

In my experience, a minute of true rapport is worth more than an hour of collecting facts. In that minute, in a flash of empathic understanding, you may suddenly see the 'centre of the case'. With more experience, you will sometimes know what the patient's remedy is during these special moments in time. This does not mean that you prescribe that remedy without further ado. You will still need to check that the remedy in mind really fits the case.

A homeopathic student of mine, an experienced general practitioner, presented an excellent example of this type of sudden rapport to a group of doctors studying homeopathy. Unfortunately, the case had been taken before she had started studying homeopathy. Nevertheless the fact that it had stayed in her mind and she had felt the need to talk about it in this homeopathic supervision group is significant. (Many homeopaths eventually suffer from the frustration of suddenly intuitively knowing what remedy a person needs – a few years too late!)

A married couple whose marriage was in serious trouble had consulted her for help. I found her account of the consultation so moving and useful that I asked her to recount it on tape. Here is her unedited transcript of her description of what transpired in the short, standard general practice, consultation:

Homeopathic doctor in supervision group: The consultation was a normal GP consultation. Husband and wife came in. The wife did all the talking initially and said that she had decided she couldn't live with her husband any longer. He was stifling her by his neediness and so she was going to leave him but she was worried that this had put him into a suicidal state and could I sort it out please?

So already at this stage I was feeling intensely irritated and cross by the wife and the man who hadn't even uttered a word at this moment, and was thinking that I was going to tell them to go to Relate and to leave me alone, basically. But because she mentioned suicide I again crossly thought that at least I would have to assess the man's risk but I was feeling so irritated and angry by the whole situation, it started to set off alarm bells in my head. That made me do something I do in that situation when I'm feeling that I'm really in my stuff and not in the patient's and I said a little prayer that I say to myself which is "Your eyes please?" It is my way of saying "Can I see this person as You would see him?" So without all my stuff getting in the way, and almost immediately, there was a very big change in the energy in the room from my point of view and I immediately felt a lot more centred in myself. I looked up at this man and instead of feeling this intense irritation towards him that I'd felt before, I could just see a really frightened person sitting there, which opened me up to compassion instead of irritation, so suddenly I was present for this guy and not trying to throw him out the room.

I then, for no obvious reason, it was just the question that came straight into my mind, asked "Could you tell me about your parents' marriage?"

This guy was still very defensive, very cross-legged, sitting back grumpily, sort of saying "I don't see how that's relevant."

So I said "Well, could you tell me anyway, I'd like to know something about it, it may be relevant" and he said "As far as I know it was happy" and all his answers were very monosyllabic and closed, closing me off more really but because I wasn't reacting to that. I was still in my sort of inquiring, gentle space, I suppose. I pursued and just gently carried on with the questioning and said "You say it was happy, are your parents still alive?" to which he just said "No, my father's dead, he died when I was 12".

I said "Well that was very long ago, it must have been very difficult for you, do you know what happened?"

"He committed suicide"

So I said "That must have been an awful thing, can you tell me some more about that?"

And there were all these very long silences before my questions. I always wait a bit, he was not forthcoming at all, and he then told me how he'd come home from school and found his father hanging in the kitchen, and again he just sort of stopped dead after telling me that, there was no emotion, still folded arms, quite dispassionate, so I was obviously quite shocked to hear it. I can remember not feeling shocked at the time, I was kind of still fine with it, so I said, "How old was your father?" and he said "44" and I said "how old are you?" again, with long pauses in between each question, and he said "44" and I said "Are you frightened you won't make 45?" at which stage he completely… he just started sobbing and sobbing and sobbing and it all just sort of, big release and after he'd sobbed for quite a long time… it then all came out, the story, of how he'd found his Dad, how that day he hadn't come straight home from school, he'd disobeyed his parents, he'd gone to play football with his friends in the park and if only he hadn't done that, if he'd come straight home from school, he might have got there early enough and how this sense of it that it had all been his fault for being this disobedient child… and he then told me about a recurrent nightmare that he had, where he, it was never about his father, that situation, he said the situations were different every time but it was always the same ending, and the ending of the nightmare was that he was always just too late and so, I wasn't doing homeopathy at that time so I didn't have a remedy to give him, nor knowledge of a remedy but it was just sort of real outpouring within about… a normal GP conversation 15 minutes… it was getting right to the centre of the case in a very short space of time, in a very intense exchange somehow but it was all created by this extra energy that somehow came from somewhere else when I got out of my space, it kind of liberated up a lot of room for things to happen in…"

Brian Kaplan (as supervisor): Somehow you were able to see the case without the filtration of your own ego, own personality.

Homeopathic doctor: Yes, definitely, and it almost felt like I wasn't me, because normally I'm quite an emotional person but I can remember feeling very calm and very able to handle what he was telling me…

She now knew that:

- the husband, as well as feeling suicidal, was fearful of death rather than angry

- he was keeping the fear hidden behind a mask of passive aggression and had probably not talked to anyone about it

- he had suffered a significant grief in his life which had probably also been suppressed

- he felt guilty and irrationally responsible for his father's death.

If she had been even a beginner homeopath at the time, this information would obviously be central to a homeopathic prescription. (Natrum muriaticum came to her mind on reflecting on the case although other remedies such as Aurum metallicum also come into consideration. A few questions about general symptoms and physical complaints would probably make the choice of remedy clear.)

All this crucial information became available in a second. It was not the length of the consultation that produced it, but the change in the doctor when she said to herself: "Your eyes, please?" I do not know the religion of this student and I did not ask her as it is not important because the actual words of her prayer are clearly non-denominational. What she had asked or prayed for was simply to be without prejudice. Her little prayer had worked and for one glorious moment she had managed to eliminate herself and her ego from the process. For an instant she was able to be totally objective rather than subjective. In that instant everything was clear and she knew that she had made a quantum leap in her understanding of the case. This was a wonderful breakthrough in the consultation. At times like this, we homeopaths feel truly at ease with ourselves and we understand what it is to be of service in our profession.

When this student mentioned 'Your eyes please?', I recalled a reference to God in a verse of a poem by Louis MacNeice.

> God or whatever means the Good
> Be praised that time can stop like this,
> That what the heart has understood
> Can verify in the body's peace
> God or whatever means the Good.
>
> *(from Meeting Point by Louis MacNeice)*[65]

The poem, which I recommend is read in its entirety, is about the meeting of a man and a woman in a coffee shop. The rapport is so strong that time seems to stand still for them. This is a true 'meeting point' and is not that different from the moment when my student suddenly understood the case above. I like MacNeice's phrase, 'God or whatever means the Good'. It is spiritual without referring to any specific religion. This is the feeling I get about Hahnemann's attitude to religion and homeopathy when reading certain passages in the *Organon*.

So how do we create this quality time in our consultations? For me it is necessary to allocate sufficient time to every consultation to allow for the possibility of these special moments. If you spend two hours on the initial consultation, you are probably more likely to share some quality time with your patient than if you allocate half-an-hour for this vital, first appointment. Probably, but not definitely. It all depends on you and your state of mind while you are consulting.

I have worked as a homeopathic doctor in the outpatients department of a busy hospital with, at most, ten minutes a consultation. However, early in my career, I had many quiet days where I only had three or four patients to consult. On these days I chose to spread the cases over the whole day to give me the luxury of having some very long consultations. At present I choose to allocate an hour for the first visit – unless the patient has travelled a very long distance to see me and there will be a big gap between the first and second appointments. If at the end of the first consultation, I feel that I have not received enough information for whatever reason, I always ask the patient to return soon for another hour's consultation. If the patient senses that this suggestion has been made totally for his own good, he will not resent this. In fact I have seen patients sigh with relief when they hear me suggest this.

Some patients will not take kindly to being asked to return for another visit without a medicine having been prescribed. There are different ways of dealing with this. You can be frank and tell them you are unsure of what to do and need to get to know them better before you can prescribe for them. I sometimes say that I will analyse the case on computer (which I do as well!) but will need to check the results of my computer analysis with them before I could think of giving them a medicine.

I prefer seeing patients for an hour at a time. People are used to a 'professional hour' of anyone's time and sometimes the case becomes clear in less than an hour. What would I have done with my infuriated Nux vomica patient for another two hours when after less than ten minutes I knew that I had to prescribe that remedy as the first prescription?

The homeopath Jeremy Sherr (head of the Dynamis School and famous for proving Scorpion, Oxygen, Chocolate and many other remedies), recently gave a masterclass for the Homeopathic Physicians Teaching Group. I interviewed him for 40 minutes about provings and homeopathy in general but inevitably asked him about receiving the case. His reply was profound and elegantly expressed. As the interview was videotaped, here is an exact transcript of what he said:

Brian Kaplan: It's almost the elimination of other things. Sometimes the patient may say something, or make you think of something in your own life but it's important to rather stay with what the patient says next rather than to tangentially go off because people will give triggers to you that will provoke emotional experiences in yourself.

Jeremy Sherr: It's about letting go, I find it's about letting go of the desire... look I have an exercise... to me homeopathic case-taking is like my best form of meditation, that's why I don't bother meditating, because for me every case-taking is an exercise in meditation like a Japanese tea ceremony. How to do it and stay centered and stay loose and stay relaxed but yet do it and be there at the same time, like t'ai chi. How to be tight and loose at the same time. And more so for me because I do video clinics. In these video clinics I have 40 people sitting in the room or next door, wanting to see how Jeremy will do the case or find a remedy, and of course that puts a whole other pressure on me. Within one hour I've got to come up with something useful and interesting and hopefully curative to the patient. So, it's a different ball game. And for me, that's even a better meditation, because I have to let go of that pressure in order to do it properly and not care. Not care but not in an indifferent way, just not get caught up that I have to go and provide... if it doesn't happen, it's not going to happen. And the bottom line of that whole thing for me is faith. Having faith that things will turn out the best way that they need to turn out, that I'll get the symptom, that the remedy will come, if it doesn't need to come, what can I do? Just do my best in every case and have the faith that things will work out well.

I love the way Jeremy compares the homeopathic consultation to meditation or a Japanese tea ceremony. It implies reverence and stillness, qualities all health practitioners should aspire to.

The ideal homeopathy for me would be to see patients weekly for an hour, much like a counsellor or psychotherapist. I would make a prescription when I had a strong 'gut feeling' for a certain remedy based on the continuing conversation and case analysis. I think it is ridiculous that we put ourselves under any sort of pressure at all to find a patient's remedy during the first consultation, whatever time we allocate for it. The patient may need some time to think about you and whether he trusts you enough to talk about his most vulnerable areas. On many occasions patients have said to me things like: 'last time when you asked me about my sex life, I said things were okay, but…' They may have not been ready to talk about sex or some other sensitive area with a perfect stranger. As a week passes and they think about you and the consultation, they may realise that it might well be in their interest to be more honest with you during the second consultation. This is a vital point to grasp. If you find it difficult to ask a patient to return for a second visit before prescribing a remedy, I suggest you have a little chat with any counsellor or psychotherapist about time. You will hear that a single hour or consultation is considered just the start of a process which may comprise an hour a week for 6 to 12 weeks (brief therapy) or several times a week for several years (psychoanalytic psychotherapy). And these professionals are not obliged to prescribe a homeopathic remedy! If we know the power of the constitutional remedy, why should we restrict the time we spend on trying to find it? The only alternative is to prescribe placebo or give the patient a remedy that we are somewhat unsure about. What would you want for yourself if you were the patient? It's a rhetorical question, isn't it?

The amount of time we spend with patients is a highly individual matter. It is up to you how much time you spend with each patient and how many patients you see in a day. I am aware that many of you will not have much flexibility in this. You can only do your best under the circumstances. If you work in a system where you have to see many patients every day, then don't hesitate to bring them back for several consultations before prescribing. If you are tempted to shorten your consultation times to earn more money, I would suggest you think again about it. In saying this, it is the quality of your life that I am thinking about, as well as that of your patients!

I would like to leave the final word about time to Jiddu Krishnamurti. It was after listening to him speak and reading transcripts of his discourses that I began to have an inkling of an understanding of the relationship between thought, memory, consciousness and time.

> To put it very simply, when you want to understand something, what is the state of your mind? When you want to understand your child, when you want to understand somebody, something that someone is saying, what is the state of your mind? You are not analysing, criticising, judging what the other is saying; you are listening, are you not? Your mind is in a state where the thought process is not active but is very alert. That alertness is not of time, is it? You are merely being alert, passively receptive and yet fully aware; and it is only in this state that there is understanding. When the mind is agitated, questioning, worrying, dissecting, analysing, there is no understanding. When there is the intensity to understand, the mind is obviously tranquil. This, of course, you have to experiment with, not take my word for it, but you can see that the more and more you analyse, the less and less you understand. You may understand certain events, certain experiences, but the whole content of consciousness cannot be emptied through the analytical process. It can be emptied only when you see the falseness of the approach through analysis. When you see the false as the false, you begin to see what is true; and it is the truth that is going to liberate you from the background.[66]

The length of time spent in consultation is not nearly as important as the amount of time spent with the type of receptivity described here. In the context of homeopathy, it is hardly surprising that quality is more important than quantity.

Chapter 12

Children

What can one say about talking to children? It helps to have children of your own, but not that much. Children and babies are as different from each other as adults. Obviously, they have shorter life stories and this does make things a little easier for the homeopath. On the other hand there are many additional skills homeopaths need to learn in order to have meaningful conversations with children.

The whole area of treating children in homeopathy is in need of much more attention. The big problem is that all the provings were carried out on adults so we do not have very good drug pictures for children. The information we do have about treating children is based on clinical experience. One of the most useful children's remedies of all, Carcinosin, was developed by Dr Donald Foubister, purely on what he had observed in his paediatric outpatient clinic at the Royal London Homoeopathic Hospital. Paul Herscu's excellent book, *The Homeopathic Treatment of Children*,[67] is essentially a materia medica of just eight, very useful, constitutional remedies for children. The book is full of examples of homeopathic diagnoses made on observations as well as symptoms.

Clearly the homeopathic world needs more literature on the treatment of children. If a child has clear symptoms that can be repertorised, we can prescribe the indicated remedy, but this does not obviate the need for comprehensive materia medica for children. It is highly likely that any remedy useful in adults is also going to be helpful for children. We need to know what types of children respond to the various remedies. We also need to learn how to talk to children in order to elicit reliable, homeopathic data.

Children's emotional response to being ill is likely to be learnt from their parents and carers. A child whose mother gets very anxious at every cold and cough may well copy this parental response and learn to be anxious himself every time he falls ill. Therefore it is worth being aware of the attitude of the parents to help you assess what the child might be experiencing. When you speak to the parents, watch the child's response to the talking parent. Is there increased anxiety, irritation or perhaps nonchalance towards the parent?

Children are highly sensitive and susceptible to their environments. Their physical health may be affected by stressful events such as divorce, bereavement, sibling rivalry, moving home or financial problems. Chronic illnesses are more common when stress is ongoing and sometimes it may be necessary to counsel the family about this in order to help the child.

Neonates and babies

The first-born is generally the hardest to treat as you have no frame of reference within the family. Additionally, first-time parents might have increased anxiety about their child's health, which then gets passed on to the child. If the child is not the first-born, I always ask: 'What is he like compared to his brother/sister at the same age?' My experience has been that all parents are aware of personality differences between their children almost from the moment they are born. The differences they notice can provide valuable homeopathic information.

In his classic text, *Birth Without Violence,* Frederik Leboyer [68] gives the reader an idea of what it feels like to undergo the traumatic journey of birth itself. You start off in an idyllic environment of gentle shades of light, floating and moving effortlessly in soothingly warm, amniotic fluid. And then! Well, I recommend you read the book for the details. Suffice to say that things start to get progressively less comfortable. Finally the journey ends and you enter a very different world indeed! For many years this used to be a world of harsh lights and rough towels. Fortunately, thanks to the efforts of Leboyer, Odent and others, things have improved in recent years. This is true of England and France and especially Holland, where approximately a third of all babies are born at home.

Leaving the uterus can be a very bruising journey. If forceps or ventouse are used, the bruises on the neonate are all too apparent. In these cases a dose of Arnica is a good idea.

I believe that all mothers should be given a dose of Arnica after childbirth for the unavoidable internal bruising. If there has been an episiotomy or Caesarean section, a dose of Staphisagria is often helpful. The body 'resents' being cut in this way even if the mother has come to terms with it psychologically. This physical 'resentment' is the reason why Staphisagria has such a good reputation in the treatment of incised wounds.

I always talk to new-born children. Even though they are pre-verbal, they are very sensitive to the feelings behind the words. It is important to speak to them in an open, honest and friendly way. The baby is sensitive to the actions and emotions of the homeopath, so keep in mind Rogers' qualities of authenticity, empathy and warmth. It certainly isn't too much of a challenge to feel warmth towards a new-born child. They stare at you with such unconditional trust and are so non-judgemental that it is hard not to love them at all.

The oversight we can make with babies is to forget the necessity of building a relationship between homeopath and patient. The temptation is to relate only to the parents. This is a very natural error as they are the ones who do the talking. It is necessary to reassure the parents and explain what you are trying to achieve with homeopathy – but don't forget the baby!

Children

Observational skills are obviously important when seeing children and babies. Observation should start in the waiting room and continue until the child leaves the consulting room. I often get interesting feedback from my reception about how the child relates to his mother or which toys he chooses. It is worth noting how the child relates to its parents. Is it clingy or striving for independence? Demanding or accepting? A toy box in the consulting room is essential. Dr Anne Wynne-Simmons in the *The Children's Toy Box,* [69] a handy booklet, gives a lot of useful information on how different babies and children relate to various toys.

The current homeopathic literature based on detailed observation is useful but more information is needed on conversing with children in the homeopathic context. I hope that books on this subject will be written by homeopathic paediatricians, of which there far too few at present. It is a great pity that child psychiatrists are not generally interested in homeopathy. All classical homeopaths are aware of the incredible behavioural changes effected in 'difficult children' by a single dose of remedies such as Stramonium, Hyoscyamus and Tuberculinum.

Didier Grandgeorge's book, *The Spirit of Homeopathic Medicines*,[70] is essentially a materia medica but includes many illustrative cases. A good proportion of these involve children and babies and much can be learned from his conversations with them and their parents .

Here are a few tips I have picked up over the years about talking to children.

Get down to the level of the child
I mean physically, of course! As the child enters your room, get down on your knees so that your face is at the same level as theirs. We all know what it feels like to speak up at someone who is much taller than we are.

Observe the child carefully
What you hear in the consulting room may not tally with what you observe. For example, an ADHD (attention deficit hyperactivity disorder) child will not necessarily display hyperactive behaviour in the consulting room as these children tend to function much better when only required to relate to one person.

Speak softly
This was taught to me by an optometrist and has proved to be invaluable advice. Children and babies have sensitive hearing and a loud voice, however friendly, can be disconcerting. Of course, if the child has a hearing difficulty (most cases are due to 'glue ear'), you will have to adjust your voice accordingly. In these cases it is essential to maintain a gentle tone – which takes a little practice.

Make some form of physical contact
Stroke a baby's face and shake hands with children. If they try to avoid this, note it down as a homeopathic symptom. On the other hand children who want to hug you or sit on your lap often need a dose of Phosphorus.

Respect the child
Children will sense if you are being patronising, speaking down to them or talking to their parents and excluding them from the conversation. They need you to be kind and to explain to them what's going on and what might happen. Finally, they need you to be honest with them. Do not underestimate the psychological effect of reassurance.

Ask simple questions
Be very direct and simplify your language. You may need to say something like: 'I would like to help you get better and we need to find a good medicine

for you. I need to understand you so I am going to ask lots of questions but this is not like school where you give me a right or wrong answer. Just say whatever you want.'

We should try to avoid closed questions with yes or no answers. For younger children we can ask questions with choices which include a third, open option, or allow the child to answer affirmatively to both options if need be: 'When you are in bed do you like lots of cuddles or do you like to be on your own, or is there something else you like to do?'

Children will talk about what they are familiar with. Instead of 'Do you like school?' (expecting a certain response) we can ask, 'What's your favourite thing at school?' and 'What do you hate most at school?' These very simple questions allow the child to answer honestly without betraying anyone. Such questions can also elicit all sorts of useful information.

The child needs to know he is understood and the right question will help you both by engendering trust in the child and helping you acquire relevant material. By asking questions that also legitimise 'bad' behaviour, the child will relax and feel that you understand him. Here are some examples:

'Do you have any pets at home? Do you like animals?'

'Do you get on with your little sister, and share your toys, or do you get annoyed if she takes them away while you are playing?

'Do you ever get so angry you want to hit her?

'Do you ever get bullied at school, or are you the one that does the bullying?'

'When you get upset, do you run away and hide, or do you shout and scream and throw your toys about?'

Listen to the child's view of his illness
While speaking to a child, listen to his voice and his concerns. Children can be quite intuitive and understanding of their illnesses. You can ask some children for an interpretation of the illness. In answer to a question like: 'Why do you think you get asthma?', they may give you a useful psychosomatic link like: 'I usually get it after I get on the school bus and say goodbye to Mummy'.

Teenagers
From adolescence some children might need, or prefer, a consultation without their parents. As well as giving them my card, I offer e-mail contact and offer them the opportunity to contact me independently.

Challenging cases
If there are severe emotional and behavioural difficulties, I always ask the parents for any assessments the child might have had. These might include annual school reports or a statement of special educational needs including reports from psychologists, speech and language therapists, audiologists, occupational therapists and so on. I may also suggest assessments myself. One of the most useful tools is an art therapy assessment. Many children enjoy painting and drawing and some will find it easier to show in pictures what is happening to them. In art therapy the child is not under pressure to communicate with words or to answer questions, but can spontaneously express what he is feeling.

I remember a case of a six-year-old girl with behavioural problems. I had taken the homeopathic history from the child and her mother but was undecided between Lachesis, Stramonium, Belladonna and Hyoscyamus. The mother accepted my suggestion of an art therapy assessment. In the assessment, the child produced several images which were sexually precocious and exhibitionistic. I was then able to prescribe Hyoscyamus with confidence and she did very well.

Give the child your card
I often give my card to children from the ages of eight or nine at the same time as giving a card to their parents. I explain to the child that it is good to speak to their parents about their problems but there may come a time when they wish to speak to me privately. I have found that both child and parents invariably appreciate this. Most children do not make use of this card but some do, perhaps encouraged by their parents.

See children once a year at least
Even if the child is completely 'cured' ask them to come back for an annual 'check-up'. This conversation is worth its weight in Aurum metallicum. Children grow up so fast and change so much that our relationship with them is vulnerable. An annual visit helps us keep in touch with their lives. This is especially true just before, during and after adolescence where the child goes through a rollercoaster of physical and psychological changes.

I would like to relate a case where I learnt just this, and more. A boy whom I had treated very successfully up to the age of 13 did not return for four years. His mother attended the consultation as she always had in the past. Unfortunately for me I did not appreciate that at 17 he was quite a different person from the one I thought I knew. I was friendly and chatted to him about the subjects he was studying at school and the sports he was involved in. I prescribed a remedy on a few useful keynotes. A few weeks later I was astounded and dismayed to receive a letter from his mother saying how disappointed he had been with the consultation. Apparently I had not listened to what he really wanted to talk about and I had spoken about subjects that were of more interest to me than to him. He had been 'too polite' to interrupt me. (And too shy to write to me himself, I ascertained.) Now they were considering looking for a new homeopath. As I read the letter I felt a mixture of disappointment, anger and self-criticism. Nevertheless I decided to do something about it. I wrote a letter addressed to both mother and son, apologising for not listening properly. However I asked them to take into consideration that in the four years since I had last seen him, the boy I had known had become a young man. I said that I would quite understand if he wanted to choose another homeopath. I would be prepared to recommend someone else and send them a copy of my case notes if that was what they wanted. Within a week I received a letter from the mother thanking me for my letter and accepting my apology. She said that she and her son had read my letter and now felt much better about what had happened. They thought it generous of me to be prepared to hand over the case to another homeopath, but had decided to retain me as their homeopathic doctor.

This case was very instructive for me. The correspondence in writing proved to be of immense value. The mother had probably expected me to take a defensive position and perhaps not even bother to reply to her letter. My letter of apology, which also pointed out mitigating circumstances for my behaviour during the consultation, was well received. I believe this was because the letter was carefully written with warmth and understanding and was certainly genuine. It had taken me over an hour to write it but this was time well spent. I later realised that the correspondence between us had simply been a homeopathic conversation in itself, albeit a much more authentic conversation than the one that had taken place in my consulting room. Looking at the correspondence homeopathically, I realised that I had gained a lot of useful information about the young man:

- He was sensitive and quite shy

- He was a closed rather than open person

- He was easily hurt emotionally

- Having been hurt emotionally, he would choose to end a relationship, even though that relationship had been fine for many years

- He was sensitive to the feelings of others. When he realised how apologetic I had felt about the consultation, he sympathised with me and also realised that I cared for him more than he had thought.

I did not have to think very long about the whole episode to make a prescription of Natrum muriaticum. This is just another illustration of how observation of a patient's behaviour is often more reliable than their descriptions of themselves. When a patient is angry or dismayed with you, don't think about yourself and your ego and become defensive. Think about them and see the homeopathic symptoms acted out in front of your eyes. It's a tough lesson to learn because we feel hurt when we do our best and get criticised and attacked. But how else would you expect a patient needing Nitric acid to act?

I consider it a great privilege to treat children. I have now treated some children from birth to 18. These young adults are usually the easiest patients to treat. This is not surprising because: I have known them all their lives; I have genuine affection for them; and they have had time to build up trust in me over the years. This is the beauty of homeopathy. We can watch our patients over the years and decades, congratulate them when they succeed and help them with homeopathy when they stumble. There is an affection that can exist between patient and doctor or homeopath that is appropriate and entirely confined to the consulting room. It is an emotion that every doctor has felt for a patient at the very moment he realises what it means to be trusted totally by that patient.

The public is rightly outraged when this trust is breached in any way and this is why doctors were obliged to take the Hippocratic Oath for many years. I have mentioned the oath before and I am deliberately drawing your attention to it again. It has much to say about the doctor-patient relationship and is unequivocal about what is permissible and what is not. I have a copy of it in my consulting room and read it every now and then. I don't do this to keep me on the straight and narrow but to remind myself of how fortunate I am to belong to such a noble profession. Since specialising in homeopathy, the oath has become even more significant to me. Hippocrates was an holistic physician if ever there was one.

Children need to be able to trust their doctors and homeopaths unconditionally. Sometimes, especially in their teens, they will tell us things they would not dream of telling their parents, especially regarding sexual matters. Doctors and health professionals are privileged to be trusted in this way. To watch a child slowly develop into an adult can be a wondrous experience. To be able to be of some help during this crucial transition is a very great privilege for anybody. It is my experience that we and our remedies can indeed be of help to children. It is a position of great responsibility; but that is what being a homeopath is all about.

Chapter 13

Other Homeopaths

How many homeopaths do you know who are sure of their own constitutional remedy? Not many, I am sure. Those homeopaths who are aware of their constitutional remedy are usually those who decided to study homeopathy precisely because they were so impressed with the effect of having that remedy prescribed for them. It is common knowledge that it is difficult to get good homeopathic treatment if you are a homeopath yourself. This is very unfortunate as it is not necessarily true of other forms of holistic medicine such as acupuncture and naturopathy.

In my opinion the reason it is difficult to prescribe for other homeopaths is that homeopathic prescriptions are based on words. A symptom is the description by the patient of a bodily or mental sensation that he perceives as deviating from health. In order to describe this subjective experience, he has to use words. Unfortunately for the homeopath who is a patient, he is fully aware of which words, phrases and sentences will make an impact on the homeopath who is taking his case. He knows, for example, that if he admits to a fear of darkness, this will be considered as important information in the analysis of his case. He cannot prevent himself deciding on how much emphasis to use when talking about this fear and every other symptom. Thus a process of subtle filtration of information occurs before it is presented to the homeopath taking the case. I have called this process a 'loss of innocence'.

The patient who is also a homeopath is simply not able to describe his symptoms or answer questions with the simple innocence of a patient who has no knowledge of homeopathy. A patient can give you the priceless gift of a rare and peculiar symptom without realising he has said anything of the slightest importance. A homeopath, or even a student of homeopathy, is unable to do this because of his knowledge and understanding of homeopathy.

This seems so unfair. An acupuncturist has a much better chance of receiving effective acupuncture than a homeopath of getting an accurate prescription. This is because acupuncture uses specific signs such as the pulse and the state of the tongue to make diagnoses whereas homeopaths must rely mainly on symptoms. Signs, being objective, are more reliable than symptoms which tend to be more subjective.

Of course we can try to prescribe for ourselves but I am afraid that it is even more stupid for a homeopath to treat himself than for a lawyer to defend himself in court. The lawyer may occasionally win his case but the homeopath who treats himself almost inevitably has 'a fool for a patient'. The truth is that we are incapable of seeing ourselves as others see us. Taking the case, analysing the case and choosing a remedy requires objectivity. We simply cannot be objective enough about ourselves to do any of these tasks well enough to treat ourselves effectively. So what can we do about this?

When a homeopath comes to see you, it is important to regard it as a great compliment. He obviously knows other homeopaths and has chosen you among many for a reason. Perhaps he admires the way you think homeopathically or is in awe of your encyclopaedic knowledge of materia medica. Perhaps you are simply someone he feels he can really trust. When a homeopath consults me, I always remind myself how long it took me to receive a remedy that was clinically effective. I also remember how frustrating it was to take remedies that were no help at all while in my practice I was making some very effective prescriptions for my patients.

Initially I listen to the homeopath's story in the normal way without interruption. However I am also listening carefully for the right time to digress. My aim is to engage the homeopath in a conversation that has apparently nothing to do with homeopathy or a description of himself. I try to get him to talk freely about any subject he feels passionate about. Then I will deliberately try to provoke him in some way, using the techniques described in Chapter 10. My aim is to elicit reliable responses there and then in the consulting room rather than rely on words that have been unconsciously filtered by a mind educated in homeopathy.

A favourite method of provocation is to ask the homeopath whether he has prescribed a remedy for himself. If he has done this – and most homeopaths have – I may then choose to mock the choice of remedy, suspecting that it did not act, otherwise why would he be consulting me? If he has not prescribed for himself for some time, I ask him what he thinks his constitutional remedy might be. Whatever he says I laugh at, pointing out the reasons why it is a ridiculous choice. I may do this even if he mentions a remedy I am seriously considering giving him. I may suddenly and apparently inappropriately ask him intimate questions about his sex life. All the time I am watching his responses to my attempts at provocation and trying to be as sensitive as possible to the atmosphere in the room. My aim is to provoke him to act out his remedy right there in front of my desk! This may take a number of consultations but homeopaths tolerate this as they know how easy it is to prescribe a remedy but how hard it is to prescribe one that will have any effect.

If I sense that the homeopath is beginning to become comfortable with this unusual type of conversation and even tease me back a little, I may then choose to start asking 'boring' homeopathic questions about temperature preferences, food desires and aversions and standard enquiries about anxieties and fears in a serious voice that is obviously contrived. Here there is a chance of catching him off guard and getting some 'unfiltered' answers. There is method in this madness and it can be quite enjoyable. As long as you remember at all times what a compliment your patient is paying you in choosing you as his homeopath, I think it is quite ethical to make the most outrageous comments or ask the most ridiculous questions, all in the name of indirectly eliciting useful homeopathic information.

If you feel incapable or unwilling to talk to a fellow homeopath like this you may have to try to help your patient in other ways. Before I started to try the provocative methods I have described, I used to advise homeopaths to consult traditional Chinese acupuncturists or healers in other disciplines, but there is one other way of trying to locate the right remedy for a patient who is a classical homeopath himself. You can advise the homeopath to consult another homeopath who is also a trusted, personal friend of his. Even if this friend is fairly inexperienced as a homeopath, he will have had the advantage of observing your patient in everyday life and this could make a crucial difference in his ability to assess the patient. This is how I was first prescribed an effective remedy myself. A good friend who is an excellent classical homeopath living in a different country, agreed to take my case. I was happy for him to talk to my wife who inevitably contradicted some of my own views about myself. In the end he prescribed a remedy that had a very good effect.

'What was the remedy?' I can hear you asking. Now let me give you some advice about homeopathic ethics. In my opinion it is unethical to ask a patient any question simply out of curiosity when you are pretty sure that the answer is not going to give you any useful homeopathic information. However it is quite ethical to ask your patient any question if there is a reasonable chance that his response will help you locate his remedy. Telling you what remedy acted on me will not improve your homeopathic skills so I am not going to tell you what it is. I refuse to allow you to indulge in any voyeuristic tendency you might have.

I hope that you were at least *slightly* provoked by the previous paragraph. Now answer the following multiple choice question:

Do you call yourself

a) a psychopath?
b) an allopath?
c) a homeopath?
d) a homoeopath?
e) a homœopath?

If you consider yourself to be a *classical* prescriber then the most correct answer is *e)* a homœopath. The diphthong 'œ' originates from classical Greek so it has to be the best answer. *d)* a homoeopath is a reasonable answer especially if you don't know how to type 'œ' on a keyboard but *c)* a homeopath is an unacceptable way of describing a classical homœopath.

By the way, I am particularly interested in how you describe yourself on your letterheads and cards and not how you chose to answer the question on the spur of the moment. If you are using the absolutely unacceptable term 'homeopath', I suggest you change all your stationery and cards and substitute the correct term 'homœopath' Do it now, before you read another word of this book!

Okay, okay, I know I have used the modern spelling 'homeopath' in this book. Editors, publisher, search engines and the 21st century persuaded me to do so. I'm still a classical homœopath inside and emotionally attached to the classical spelling of the word, homœopathy. As for authors, like Julian Winston, who write magnificent books like *The Faces of Homœopathy*[71] and retain the diphthong – I admit that I harbour a secret envy of their resistance to compromise.

I hope you are getting some idea of the provocative style of homeopathic conversation. It's tough to treat other homeopaths, but what they say in the classics is also true of classical homeopathy: 'When the going gets tough, the tough get going!'

Chapter 14

Doctors and Scientists

If a medical doctor consults you as a homeopath you can be sure you have a challenging case at hand. By 'doctor' I mean a conventionally trained, orthodox physician who is not particularly interested in 'alternative' or 'complementary' medicine. We can include orthodox, paramedical professionals such as physiotherapists and scientists (of subjects such as chemistry, physics and biology) in the same general rubric. Most of these people believe in medical science and there is no way they can get their minds around the perplexing, homeopathic issue of potentisation. I have described the mechanistic approach to health and illness taught at medical school in Chapter 1. The human body is seen as a sophisticated machine. When it breaks down in some way it needs to be fixed by anatomical intervention (surgery), physiological intervention (the chemistry of orthodox medication) or replacement of something in which the body is deficient (for example hormones, vitamins, minerals and blood).

The scientist's view of a homeopathic remedy is that of putting a drop of medicine at one end of a large, swimming pool and drinking a teaspoon of the water at the other end. Homeopathic remedies, being diluted beyond Avogadro's number (6.0225×10^{-23}) can contain no molecules of the original substance and are therefore surely incapable of any physiological effect. Homeopathy must be the fine art of the placebo.

Being a doctor myself means that I get invited to various medical conferences and dinners. I seldom attend as the subject matter is usually one type of disease and the latest way of treating it with drugs or surgery. However, at one such dinner I chatted to a urologist about the problem of benign prostate hypertrophy (BPH). I listened with interest to his views about the latest drugs and how surgical intervention may be able to be avoided in the future. After 15 minutes of urological conversation without a word about Sabal serulata from myself, he finally asked me what I did for a living. I said that I specialised in homeopathy. He did not utter another word to me. Not even a polite 'good-bye'.

So why on earth would such people consult you? The answer is nearly always that someone has recommended you very strongly and they have correctly ascertained that they have little to lose by consulting you. They may have actually witnessed a marvellous improvement in the health of a relative or friend who has been treated with homeopathy. They may also be desperate. I have seen the most rabid critics of alternative medicine turn to homeopathy and other complementary therapies when told by their scientific colleagues that 'there is nothing more we can do for you'. The problem with treating doctors and other scientists is that unless you get a good response to your first prescription, they are unlikely to return at all. 'I tried homeopathy and it didn't work' is how they often describe the whole experience. Therefore it is vital to do your best to get some response to the first prescription. Of course, the best way of achieving this is to prescribe the correct constitutional remedy – but this is easier said than done!

When seeing doctors I tend to spend a long time talking about the presenting complaint and its modalities. They tend to be quite intrigued about why I am so interested in the way they experience their illness. I am cautious about talking about the mentals and generals too early in the conversation as this could lead to a rejection of the whole consultation as nonsense. Empathic interest in the details of their affliction is appreciated by most people – even doctors.

After discussing their presenting symptoms in great detail, the question: 'How does that (the symptom) leave you feeling?' does not sound so irrational and may yield some valuable information about their personality. Empathy is the key here. If you try to understand how a doctor, trained in medical science, might be feeling during the consultation, your chances of creating good rapport are much improved. If a doctor is consulting you about arthritis, questions about food desires and aversions will make no sense to him and are probably best left to the very end of the consultation. By then you may have the information you need to make a prescription. If you ask apparently 'irrational' questions too early, he might decide that homeopathy is indeed hocus pocus and lose interest in the rest of the consultation.

The consequence of this type of case-taking is that the first prescription may well be a remedy that is more suited to the main complaint and its modalities than it is to the patient as a whole. There is nothing inherently wrong with this. If you can get a small but significant improvement in the patient's symptoms, he will return. You can then afford to be a little bolder in the questions you ask and make a concerted effort at finding the constitutional remedy.

When you treat a doctor successfully, don't expect too much gratitude and don't be surprised if he attributes his improvement to something other than the homeopathic remedy prescribed. Try to understand that it is hard for him to accept that pills containing nothing could have made him better.

A young physician, suffering from Hepatitis C, consulted me many years ago. He had already consulted top physicians and virologists by the time he came to see me. I listened to his story carefully and soon became aware of how anxious and fearful he was about carrying this potentially fatal virus. I prescribed a remedy and he returned to his country far away from England. A few months later I received a picture postcard from him thanking me for seeing him and saying: 'My consultation with you was by far the most effective but I have no idea why.' I never saw him again but I continue to get cards from him announcing the birth of children and wishing me well. I would like to believe that the remedy I gave him is still keeping him well but I have no way of confirming this. What I do know is that the combination of the remedy and the homeopathic conversation has made some impact on him as a person and that so far the virus has not got the better of his immune system. Perhaps it is irrelevant whether he believes in homeopathy or not.

Doctors and medical scientists are as deserving of good homeopathic treatment as anyone else. They just need to be handled a little differently. Empathic understanding of how their view of illness and health differs from ours, is the key to creating rapport and improving your chances of making an accurate prescription.

Chapter 15

Psychotherapists and their Patients

Psychotherapists

It is hard to get a straight answer out of a psychotherapist or psychoanalyst. What you are likely to get is an *interpretation* of themselves. This is because they have all undergone analysis or psychotherapy themselves and 'worked through' their problems. What this means is that they have spent many hours talking about themselves to other psychotherapists. They are used to talking about themselves. When you ask them to say what they are like as people, you cannot be sure which person they are going to describe. The person they were before psychotherapy or the one they are now. You usually get a mixture of both.

The other problem with treating people trained in psychotherapy is that they tend to use a slightly different language when talking about themselves. They may use terms like 'denial' and 'projection'. This lingo has been described, slightly unkindly, as 'psychobabble', but I find it quite interesting and amusing. In fact I have a dictionary of these terms that I often dip into.[72] Once again empathy is the key to opening up the case. If you show some interest in their way of looking at life they are much more likely to open up to you – just as when you visit another country and make fumbling attempts to speak the language, local people tend to warm to you.

Psychotherapists have more in common with homeopaths than they do with orthodox doctors. They are more holistic in the way they understand mind, body and symptoms. A big difference between a homeopathic conversation and a session of psychotherapy is that homeopaths feel under much more pressure to do something at the end of even the first session. Psychotherapists understand how difficult it is to assess another human being in a single session. They will generally be happier than the average patient to return for a second session before receiving a prescription. When you are consulted by a psychotherapist, it is worth remembering that Hahnemann advocated 'repeated conversations' in paragraph 209 of the *Organon*.

Patients in psychotherapy

Patients who have received or who are undergoing psychotherapy have much in common with psychotherapists who have had to go through the same process as part of their training. They will also be more open to having a few conversations before receiving a remedy. This is a relief for the homeopath as it takes a lot of pressure off the first consultation.

If a patient is receiving psychotherapy at same time as coming for homeopathic treatment, it is possible to allow these two disciplines to complement each other to the obvious benefit of the patient.

If you prescribe the right constitutional remedy for a patient they may change in various ways. Physical symptoms may improve or disappear, but the patient himself may also benefit at a psychological level. This sounds good in theory and is often appreciated by people close to the patient. However it can also cause problems. Family and friends may have grown used to the ways of your patient. A sudden change in their personality could upset a certain balance in their marriage or family that everyone else has learned to live with.

A typical example of a remedy that can cause disruption is Staphisagria. A patient who has suppressed anger for years or decades might start becoming appropriately angry and self-assertive when the occasion demands it. This sudden change in attitude and behaviour can threaten important relationships in your patient's life. Their partner may even have married them because of their Staphisagria-like personality. When your patient becomes more confident and self-assertive after taking the remedy, they may find that their partner is less attracted to them or even feels threatened by them. At these times some psychotherapy and counselling can be most helpful as the patient is given time, space and encouragement to work through the internal changes they are experiencing.

Homeopathic treatment can also aid the psychotherapeutic process. A friend of mine, who is an excellent psychotherapist, seriously considered studying classical homeopathy some years ago. She had been seeing a patient for some months when the patient suddenly underwent a huge and unexpected improvement in her psychological state. My friend was not able to attribute such a sudden change to the psychotherapy so she asked her patient if anything else had happened in her life (thinking about things like falling in love or inheriting a lot of money). What had happened was that the patient had consulted a homeopath. From then on the psychotherapy became rewarding and successful for both parties. After that case, whenever she got stuck with a patient she recommended homeopathic treatment.

We had an interesting conversation about homeopathy and psychotherapy and I advised her not to train to become a professional homeopath. I told her that she was an excellent psychotherapist and good psychotherapists are hard to find. However we devised a plan where we could combine psychotherapy and homeopathy in an interesting way. When I referred her a patient, I would ask the patient how he or she felt about me talking to my friend in confidence about the case. Not a single patient objected and after a few sessions of psychotherapy we had a chat on the phone. Sometimes she would give me some extremely useful homeopathic clues that had emerged in the psychotherapy sessions and this led to some encouraging results.

After a while she began to understand what information would be most useful for me. I advised her to buy a few homeopathic books that focused on the psychological profiles of the remedies. When I thought of a few possible remedies for our mutual patient, I suggested that she read the description of the personality types of these remedies in the books I had recommended. We then had a further discussion about the patient in relation to these remedies. This proved to be very useful and much appreciated by our patients.

I was aware that this was quite an unusual approach in both of our disciplines but as the patients seemed to benefit, it seemed worthy of further exploration. Thereafter, whenever a patient told me they were undergoing psychotherapy or counselling, I asked them how they would feel about me talking to their therapist. The great majority were willing and even pleased for me to do so. I have continued to co-operate with psychotherapists and counsellors in this way and have come to the conclusion that classical homeopathy and good psychotherapy can be synergistic to the advantage of the patient.

When you talk to a patient's psychotherapist about them you are speaking to a person who has a close relationship with your patient and who has had many hours of conversation with them – something that is denied to us as homeopaths. In the final analysis it seems ridiculous not to make use of those hours of conversation in helping the homeopath find the patient's remedy.

A close homeopathic colleague of mine (my late friend Dr Lee Holland), who had been a psychiatrist before studying homeopathy, always remembered a female patient he had been unable to help as a young psychiatrist. The reason he remembered her was because when he started studying homeopathy many years later, it soon became clear to him that she was a classic case of Sepia. He could not help wondering what would have happened if he had been able to give her a dose of Sepia.

It really seems a pity that the hours spent in psychotherapy by so many patients do not result in homeopathic prescriptions. But you have to be a classical homeopath to have this regret. Perhaps homeopaths and psychotherapists can learn to work more with each other in the future.

In the case of psychoanalysis, the situation is different. The analysand and analyst meet for an hour three to five times a week and develop a very special and private relationship that is totally confidential. I do not ask patients in analysis for permission to speak to their psychoanalyst as it feels inappropriate and intrusive. However, I feel that it is quite ethical to ask patients in most forms of psychotherapy and counselling how they would feel about an approach to their therapist. Of course if the patient expresses the slightest hesitation or doubt, the matter should never be brought up again. My experience, however, is that most patients seem happy and even flattered that two professionals are prepared to spend time working together on their behalf.

Chapter 16

Non-verbal Clues, Signs and 'Symptoms'

Hahnemann's famous dictum 'similia similibus curentur' (let likes be cured by likes), stands proudly above anything else written about homeopathy. It is perhaps the one principle on which all schools of homeopathy can agree. In practical terms it means that substances capable of producing symptoms in healthy volunteers (called 'provers') are capable of curing those symptoms in patients who have a similar set of symptoms. But is this really all we homeopaths use to choose remedies for our patients?

By strict definition a symptom is something experienced subjectively by the patient, as opposed to a sign which is something seen by the doctor or homeopath. However, for all practical purposes, signs are often used as symptoms in homeopathy and it is probable that Hahnemann included them in his understanding of the word 'symptom'. Thus varicose veins, haemorrhoids that look like grapes, swollen tonsils and warts of various types, can all be considered and used homeopathically as symptoms. This is not unreasonable as the substances used to treat these signs may have been able to produce such signs in healthy volunteers.

Classical homeopaths, however, have always used much more than these symptoms and signs to prescribe remedies. How did a situation arise in homeopathy where features other than symptoms were used to prescribe remedies? Not without a huge fight – is the answer. In his under-rated book, *The Two Faces of Homoeopathy*, [73] Anthony Campbell explains how scholarly English homeopaths like Hughes and Dudgeon were much more in favour of sticking to proper symptoms (ie, symptoms that were produced in provers or appeared in toxicology studies) whereas across the Atlantic, homeopaths, in particular Kent, began to add information other than symptoms appearing in the provings to the materia medica. This information is central to almost all of the materia medicae we now use. Kent's *Lectures on Materia Medica* [74] remains a classic, whereas the books written by Hughes (in particular the scholarly A Cyclopaedia of Drug Pathogenesy [75]), Dudgeon and others are hardly read at all. I believe that the reason for this is that while the English homeopaths were scientifically correct in trying to protect the materia medica from indiscriminate additions and especially those that were not symptoms, the Americans were correct in being very vigilant in the clinic and observing what types of patients appeared to respond to the different remedies. Slowly these clinical symptoms found their way into the materia medica and are now central to most of the homeopathic drug pictures we, classical homeopaths, take for granted.

It is essential that we continue to prove new remedies and perhaps even more important to reprove old ones. It is also just as important for us to continue to be observant about what sort of patients respond to these remedies in the clinic and share this information with other homeopaths. When we start to observe patients in this way, rather than try to elicit only 'true symptoms', homeopathy tends to become even more fascinating.

We will now explore those features of patients, that although not strictly symptoms, can be extremely useful in helping us find the appropriate remedy. We will consider:

• Physical appearance

• Dress

• Body movement

• Art and images.

Physical appearance

• Blue eyes and blonde hair may encourage a prescription of Pulsatilla. I don't think you could produce these 'symptoms' in a dark-haired, brown-eyed prover if you gave Pulsatilla 10M daily to her for the rest of her life.

• Arsenicum album is said to suit fastidious people, but continuous administration of Arsenic to a man is more likely to be fatal than it is to produce a 'gentleman with a gold-headed cane'!

• Similarly, Nitric acid is said to suit 'dark-complexioned' individuals; Calcarea carbonica, the 'fat, fair, flabby'; Bryonia those of 'robust firm fibre and dark complexion'; Asterias rubens the 'flabby with red face'; Chimaphila umbellata 'women with large breasts'; and Phosphorus 'tall, slender persons, narrow chested, with thin transparent skin' (Phrases in quotes have all been taken from Boericke's *Pocket Manual of Homeopathic Materia Medica and Repertory*, a homeopathic best-seller if ever there was one. Written in 1900, it reached a ninth edition in 1927 and remains one of the most useful single-volume texts in homeopathic literature.)[76]

- The truth is that most of the materia medicae in common use are full of physical descriptions of patients that couldn't possibly have been produced by proving remedies. I see no harm in this even though it is not entirely consistent with the dictum 'similia similibus curentur'. We cannot ignore the fact that these descriptions of patients (with a predisposition to respond to certain remedies), have proved invaluable to several generations of classical homeopaths.

Dress

In a marvellous article called 'Homoeopathy a la mode', published anonymously in *Homoeopathy*, [77] Dr Marianne Harling explores the relationship of certain styles of dressing with particular homeopathic remedies. She recently confirmed in a telephone conversation with me that the article comprised information from materia medicae and the repertory in addition to her personal observations.

Here are few examples of 'sartorial symptoms' and the remedies they may indicate:

- Phosphorus: beautiful, rather than elegant, looks good in almost any clothes with a possible preference for bright reds

- Calcarea phosphorica: wears expensive clothes with elegance with the men looking best in casual clothes

- Calcarea carbonica: subdued, pastel colours, expensive clothes, lots of powder and wears clean underwear perhaps 'for the doctor'

- Arsenicum album: warm underwear (for this chilly remedy!), fussy appearance. Nevertheless Dr Harling suggests that this fussiness 'lacks the repose of true elegance'

- Nux vomica: the truly well-dressed, in a formal sense, unless you happen to see them the 'morning after'

- Ignatia: dresses like a 'drama queen' with more effort than elegance, dramatic colour combinations or, paradoxically, all in black

- Sulphur: I agree with Dr Harling that the idea of the 'ragged philosopher' is very misleading. It does occasionally apply but more often the patient wears bright clothes that often clash, and perhaps an excess of jewellery. They may obviously be trying to make an effort to look elegant but never quite pull it off. Dr Harling remarks that Sulphur will not be wearing underwear whereas Psorinum will, but this is not to be taken too seriously!

- Natrum muriaticum: Individuals needing this remedy tend to dress unadventurously and may lack colour sense. Dr Harling mentions that the men's clothes may need pressing and miss buttons

- Sepia: may wear clothes that look dingy

- Silica: are so chilly that they may be unwilling to get undressed at all for a clinical examination, whereas

- Hyoscyamus: 'wants to be naked' (Kent) so may take off all their clothes for any examination requested by the doctor. The repertory lists 'Fur, wraps up in summer'. Dr Harling wrote in 1980 that she was still waiting for the patient who visits her on a hot summer's day with nothing on under a fur coat. I believe she is still waiting.

The following phrases, found in the repertory, all refer to dress: 'Elegance, lack of; Bizarre clothes; Untidily dressed women'.

Thus in homeopathy it seems justified to judge a book by its cover but certainly the contents of the book, which is the detailed case history, should be considered much more important.

Posture and movement

The way a patient moves and sits should always be carefully noted by the homeopath. This applies to the waiting room and the consulting room. An exhibition of restlessness is a better indication for remedies such as Rhus tox. and Arsenicum album than whatever the patient may say. In my consulting room, the patient has a choice of two chairs. One is a lower-seated and comfortable armchair while the other is higher-seated, more upright and with a wooden back support. The great majority of patients choose the less comfortable chair, perhaps because it puts them at the same level as me and therefore less 'vulnerable'. However, some patients enjoy sinking into the armchair and I have yet to see a Sulphur patient choose the less comfortable chair!

Books on 'body language' are readily available and every homeopath should at least take an interest in the subject.

Art and images

I always ask patients to show me any art they have produced themselves. If they are professional artists, I request to be invited to their exhibitions.

I have very often found this to be useful in gaining new clues about the patient. A patient who is talented at producing images may reveal much more this way than in a normal homeopathic interview.

Even patients who claim that they cannot draw or paint at all may give valuable clues if asked to show the homeopath any piece of art or image of any kind that they have produced. In the case of a child this can be an invaluable way of gaining vital homeopathic information. When I am talking to the mother of a young patient, I often give the child drawing materials and ask him/her to draw something, often a picture of their family. The drawing produced, its quality being irrelevant, produces a focus for a chat with the child about important issues which could yield vital homeopathic information.

Occasionally a piece of art alone strongly suggests a specific homeopathic remedy. My wife is an art therapist and professional colleague; sometimes she is able to show me some of the images produced by her patients. Although these people are usually not homeopathic patients, it is often quite startling how some pictures can strongly suggest specific homeopathic remedies.

The following diagrams are tracings made from the artwork from one particular patient.

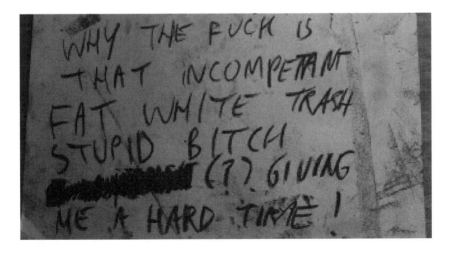

Figure 1. *This is full of swear words although the patient was asked to make images rather than write down words. The words suggest tremendous aggression and even violence. As they are also obscene, it would seem reasonable to extract the symptom 'cursing' from this 'picture'*

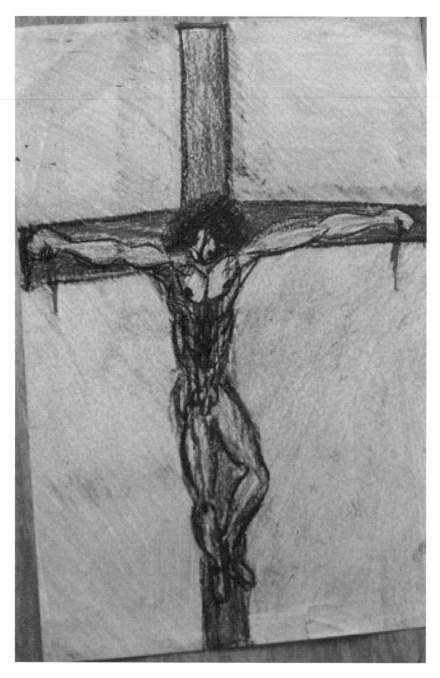

Figure 2. *This crucifixion has obvious religious significance, but the depiction of the blood and genitalia suggest a violent disposition and sexual undertones, respectively*

Figure 3. *The client has written the word 'angel' but the figure looks distinctly demonic. From a Jungian point of view this is surely a depiction of the 'shadow'. The picture shows the patient to be torn between angelic and demonic traits of his own personality*

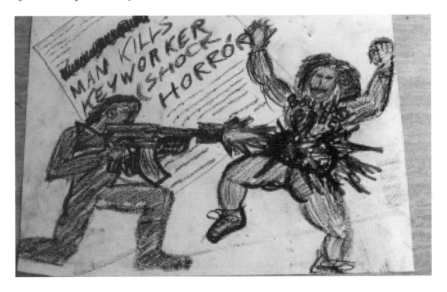

Figure 4. Considering that this picture was painted at the same session as Figure 1, it is reasonable to assume that it depicts a fantasy of the patient involving himself and his 'key worker' (the professional most responsible for his wellbeing)

The painting in Fig. 4 shows the patient shooting the female key worker with what looks like an automatic weapon. This is no spur-of-the-moment crime of passion. This is clear from the premeditated, military style positioning of the gunman. This looks more like a killing made by a hit man showing no remorse whatsoever although his victim's life is clearly portrayed as being in total disarray, still alive but surely soon to die. From this we can feel justified in using the symptom 'cruelty'.

So from the paintings alone we have:

• Cursing

• Confusion between good and bad aspects of the self (an angel on one shoulder and the devil on the other)

• religious imagery always tainted by some dark aspect

• a pervading sexuality associated more with violence rather than love.

This is enough to make a strong case for the remedy, Anacardium. When I saw that the images suggested Anacardium, I asked for more information on the case. Sure enough the patient had been diagnosed as schizophrenic and had a history of cruelty, having killed a cat. I was told that in group art therapy sessions he could be very gentle and softly spoken, also typical of the type of paradoxical personality that responds to Anacardium.

Prescriptions of homeopathic remedies are based on the patient's description of his illness in his own words. But words are only words. They are not the thing itself, which is exactly how the patient experiences his illness. Most of our patients are fairly comfortable with the medium of language. When they are asked a question, there is often time for the unconscious mind to filter the answer, with the homeopath consequently not getting the whole truth. When such patients are asked to produce an image on paper there is usually less familiarity with the medium of producing images than with the spoken word. The unconscious mind may spill itself on to a piece of paper providing the homeopath with priceless 'symptoms'.

It is clear that for many years homeopaths have been using clinical symptoms (as well as symptoms appearing in the provings) to help find the best remedies. This is no substitute for taking a homeopathic history by listening to patients in the careful, respectful and non-intrusive way long advocated by Hahnemann, Kent and all classical homeopaths. However, much information can be gained non-verbally. The general appearance of patients, the way they dress, how they move and any piece of art they have produced (or images produced by a child in the consulting room) all give valuable clues to the observant homeopath. They may even clinch the homeopathic diagnosis.

Taste in music

The effects of music on patients is well known to be useful in homeopathy. We know that patients requiring Tarentula hispanica feel better when listening to loud, rhythmical music, while those needing Natrum carbonicum may feel worse when listening to piano music.

However, it is possible to use the musical tastes of the patient in more subtle ways. I was invited to give a one-day seminar on 'Taking the Case' in Berlin recently. I took a few days off in order to sit in on the practice of my close friend and colleague, Dr Hans Zwemke, in my opinion one of the most under-rated classical homeopaths around. Hans and I spent many pleasant hours talking (and inevitably arguing) about various aspects of homeopathy and for some reason he produced a book I had never seen or heard of before. It is called *Musik in der Homoopathie* and written by the classical German homeopathic physician, Dr Sohn.[78]

This a repertory of people's reactions to music and, in this doctor's experience, the remedies that suit them. This doctor had clearly taken an interest in his patients' taste in music and made a note of what remedies they had responded to. I was really excited by this as I realised immediately that musical taste certainly individualises people and therefore should be useful in homeopathic case-taking. Just one problem: the book is only available in German which is not one of the languages I speak!

Fortunately for me, homeopathic friends tend to be good friends. Hans offered to read the whole book again and pick out a few examples that made sense to him in the context of his practice. Here are the rubrics and associated remedies selected for me by Hans Zwemke from Dr Sohn's book.

Military music (march music), likes: ars.; doesn't like: nat-m.

Pink Floyd, likes to hear music of: nux-v.

Rolling Stones, likes to hear music of: lyc., nat-m., nux-v.

Rock'n'roll, loves to dance: nat-m., puls., sep.

Musician, married to a: phos.

Verdi, likes to listen to music of: calc., lach., nat-m., phos., *sulph*
    operas of: sulph.
    Rigoletto: sulph.

Wagner, likes to hear music of: nux-v., *sulph*
    The Ring: sulph.

Fastidious, concerning music: carc., med., nux-v.

Information, listens to music to inform himself: lyc.

Slow, likes slow music-pieces: calc.

String quartets, likes to listen to: sep.

Dancing, at night on the cemetery: stram.
    nude: camph.
    half-nude: bell.

Laziness, too lazy to put on a record: sulph.

Exhaustion, sings until exhausted: tarent.

Alcoholics, singing in: cocc., op.

Answering, singing, repeats every question singing: zinc.

Anxiety, on hearing church bells: lyss.

I really enjoyed reading this selection. The image of the intellectual type of Lycopodium listening to music 'to inform himself' is hilarious but has a ring of truth about it. The idea of spouses of musicians being more likely to have a higher incidence of Phosphorus cases than the rest of us also makes a lot of sense. In fact a few such cases from my own practice immediately came to mind. It left me wanting to know more, so if you are a homeopath who understands German, I am sure you will enjoy this book. And if you enjoy yourself while you study homeopathy you will discover that your memory wasn't as bad as you thought it was!

Chapter 17

Taking Notes

> The physician advises them at the beginning of the examination to speak slowly, in order that he may take down in writing the important parts of what the speakers say.
>
> *(Organon §84)*

Of all the pieces of advice given to us by Hahnemann in the *Organon,* this is the one that has surely dated the most. I can think of no reason to ask patients to speak more slowly or faster for any reason at all. If a patient is asked to speak at a speed that does not come naturally to him, he may well use words that he would not use when talking normally. Words are of the essence in homeopathy so we may then get a somewhat distorted picture of our patient and his problem.

Of course I agree with Hahnemann that it is imperative to record all the important information the patient relates, but not at the expense of authenticity. The reason Hahnemann advised his patients to speak slowly is that it took him a long time to write down what they were saying. Perhaps this was due to the fact that he was handicapped by choosing to write with a quill which had to be dipped frequently into a bottle of ink! I have seen Hahnemann's original version of *Chronic Diseases.*[79] It is handwritten in a beautiful copperplate script. It would have been impossible for him to keep up with a patient talking at a normal pace. The homeopath of the 21st century is fortunate in that the quill has been replaced by a variety of much more user-friendly writing utensils.

If I notice a patient watching me take notes and pausing between sentences, I make a point of asking him not to worry about my notes and to speak in his normal voice. Modern homeopaths should be able to keep accurate notes without asking patients to speak slowly. Let us explore the various ways of taking notes.

Questionnaires

Some homeopaths send their patients a questionnaire to fill out before the first consultation. These questionnaires vary enormously but as a rule are restricted to routine information, such as age, address, family history, habits, previous illnesses and vaccinations. They seldom ask questions about the generals and mentals. The homeopath uses the questionnaire to save time so that he can concentrate on the more important, personal information during the first consultation.

Nevertheless he still has to read the completed questionnaire before or during the first consultation and this takes time. I have never used a questionnaire as I am curious about how a patient conveys any information to me – even his age and address. I cannot predict when the appropriate moment to ask a personal question will arrive. Some people are very sensitive about being asked their age and this sensitivity (and the reason for it) is homeopathic information. If the patient has recorded it on a questionnaire you will miss out on how he reacts to being asked his age. The same goes for previous illnesses and habits such as smoking and alcohol consumption.

My friend, colleague and fellow teacher, Dr Charles Forsyth, has kindly given me permission to include the questionnaire he has modified and developed over many years. Charles sends out this questionnaire to all new patients prior to their first visit in order to give them time to research things like family history, childhood illnesses and reactions to vaccinations. In spite of the time saved by this, he still allocates an hour for the first visit and frequently asks patients to come back for more consulting time.

This is the best homeopathic questionnaire I have ever seen and the care that has gone into its creation is obvious. Personally I choose not to use questionnaires and can neither advocate their use nor rule them out completely. It is all a matter of style and taste. The great advantage of a questionnaire is that it ensures that you get certain basic facts about your patient and you will always know where to find those facts.

REGISTRATION FORM

Date...

Title: Mr ☐   Mrs ☐   Miss ☐   Master ☐   Other...

Surname ....

Forenames .... *(Please indicate Used Forename)*

Address ....

.... Postcode.................................

Tel Home.. Tel Work ....

Fax Home... Fax Work ....

Mobile phone.. E-mail address ....

Temporary address *(if applicable)* ....

....

Postcode .... Tel ....

Date of birth .... Country of birth .... Age ....

Marital status: Married   ☐   Single   ☐   Partnered ☐

Separated ☐   Divorced ☐   Widowed ☐

Maiden name .... Religion ....

Occupations *(or previous if retired or unemployed);* school or college *(if a child or student):*

....

Spouse/partner's name .... Occupation..

Father's name .... Occupation..

Mother's name.. Occupation..

Name & initials of your family doctor (GP) ....

Address.. Postcode ....

Do you have a letter of referral from your GP? .... Yes ☐   No ☐

Would you be happy for Dr Forsyth to write to your GP?...................... Yes ☐   No ☐

Do you have Medical Insurance?

(Company name)... Yes ☐   No ☐

Do you intend to claim on your medical insurance? .... Yes ☐   No ☐

Name & initials of your specialist...

Address... Postcode ....

Do you have a letter of referral from your Specialist?........................... Yes ☐   No ☐

Would you be happy for Dr Forsyth to write to your Specialist? .... Yes ☐   No ☐

Name & initials of your osteopath/chiropractor *(if applicable)* ....

Address... Postcode ....

Do you see any other complementary therapists?

Name & initials.................................... Speciality.....................................

Address... Postcode ....

Name & initials.................................... Speciality.....................................

Address... Postcode ....

From where or whom did you obtain Dr Forsyth's name & address?
(Please give as much information as possible)

A Patient of Dr Forsyth's ☐   Another Homoeopathic Patient ☐   Your GP ☐

The British Homoeopathic Association ☐   The Faculty of Homoeopathy ☐

The Homoeopathic Development Foundation ☐   Osteopath ☐   Yellow Pages ☐

Thompson's Directory ☐   The Media ☐   A Health Food Shop ☐   A Lecture ☐

A Chemist ☐   Another Therapist ☐

Details/Other..

....

....

....

....

....

PERSONAL MEDICAL QUESTIONNAIRE

Please list briefly the main reasons, symptoms or problems (together with date of onset) that you wish to consult Dr Forsyth about:

1) ....

2) ....

3) ....

4) ....

5) ....

What other problems do you have (however minor)? Please list with dates of onset:

....

....

Please list all medications (together with dosages) that you take – whether intermittently or constantly. Include: nutritional supplements, contraceptive pill, creams, drops, lotions, suppositories, etc. When did you start taking them? ....

....

....

LIFESTYLE QUESTIONNAIRE

On how many days of the week do you drink alcohol? ....

How much alcohol do you consume per day/week? ....

How much do you smoke? .... since what age? ....

If you have now given up smoking – between what ages did you smoke? ....

how much did you smoke? ....

How much exercise do you take and in what form(s)? ....

....

How much time do you take for relaxation and what form(s)? ....

....

What are your main interests, hobbies & pastimes? ....

....

Do you suffer tiredness, fatigue or lack of energy? ....

since when? ....

What are the main stresses in your life and how do they affect you? ....

....

....

Did you have any particularly stressful or unhappy times in your childhood ? ....

....

....

....

DIETARY QUESTIONNAIRE

Are you following any special diets? (eg. vegetarian, diabetic, low fat, wholefood, high fibre, calorie controlled, macrobiotic, gluten-free, etc.) – For how long?

....

Are there any foods, drinks or drugs that upset you? In what way?

....

....

Please estimate as accurately as you can what quantity of the following you consume during an average week:

Coffee .... cups/mugs per day

Decaffeinated coffee .... cups/mugs per day

Tea .... cups/mugs per day

Soft/carbonated drinks .... glasses per week

Plain water .... glasses per week

Sugar .... teaspoons per week

Sweets & Chocolate .... quantity per week

Sweet biscuits .... number per week

Cakes .... slices per week

Puddings/desserts .... number per week

White bread .... slices per week

Wholemeal bread .... slices per week

Mammal meat (beef, pork, lamb, etc.) ...... meals per week

Poultry (chicken, turkey, etc.) .... meals per week

Fish .... meals per week

Eggs .... number per week

Cheese .... how often per week

Milk .... pints per week

Pulses (beans & lentils) .... how often per week

Fresh vegetables .... how often per week

Raw vegetables & salad .... how often per week

Fresh fruit .... quantity per week

Tinned, packeted or frozen food .... how often per week

Fast/junk food .... how often per week

How often do you add salt to your plate? ...... times per week

How often do you cook in aluminium cookware/foil? ... times per week

How many aluminium pots & pans do you have? ....

Have you ever regularly consumed food cooked in aluminium? ....
(Aluminium cooking utensils are non-magnetic and are usually dull on the cooking surface, unless they have a non-stick coating, eg Teflon).

HOUSING QUESTIONNAIRE

Approximately in which year was your house built? ....

When did you move in?...

What sort of heating do you use regularly in the winter months *(you can tick more than one)*?

Central heating: Gas ☐ Oil ☐ Coal ☐ Wood ☐ Electric ☐ Other............................

Radiators ☐ Ducted warm air ☐ Storage heaters ☐

Fires: Gas ☐ Electric ☐ Wood ☐ Coal ☐

Does the house have damp problems, mould or wet rot anywhere?.....................................

....

Do you have any pets...

....

MISCELLANEOUS

What is your Blood Group? O ☐ A ☐ B ☐ AB ☐

Rhesus: Negative ☐ Positive ☐

Are you? Dyslexic ☐ Colour blind ☐

Left handed ☐ Left footed ☐ Left eyed ☐

PAST MEDICAL HISTORY

Your Mother's pregnancy:	**IMMUNISATIONS** (Dates of each)
Your delivery:..	SMALLPOX:
At how many weeks: .... Date of Birth:	DIPHTHERIA: WHOOPING COUGH:
Induced: Rupture of membranes ☐ pessary ☐ drip ☐	TETANUS: Hib:
Forceps ☐ Ventouse ☐ Caesarian ☐	POLIO:
Penthidine ☐ Gas & Air ☐ Epidural ☐ General Anaesthetic ☐	MEASLES: RUBELLA:
Your condition at birth:..	MUMPS: MENINGITIS C
Your birth weight:	BCG (TB):
Duration breast fed:..	INFLUENZA: HEPATITIS A:
Age weaning began:...	HEPATITIS B:
Age when you first: Smiled............. Crawled............ Walked............. Talked............	CHOLERA: TYPHOID: YELLOW FEVER: RABIES:

Date	Age		Pertussis = Whooping Cough
			Triple (DPT) = Diphtheria, Pertussis & Tetanus
			Double (DT) = Diphtheria & Tetanus
			Rubella = German Measles
			IMMUNISATION REACTIONS
			DRUG SENSITIVITIES
			FOOD SENSITIVITIES
			INHALED SENSITIVITIES
			SKIN SENSITIVITIES

FAMILY MEDICAL HISTORY

Please give the year of birth and age at death of the following members of your family together with their past and present health problems, illhealth, operations, etc. Particularly relevant will be those problems that you also have or have had. Please include any of the problems listed below:

Addison's disease, Aids, Alcoholism, Allergies, Alopecia, Angina, Asthma, Birth defects, High blood pressure, Cancer, Chest trouble, Cirrhosis, Coeliac disease, Colitis, Crohn's disease, Cystic fibrosis, Dementia, Depression, Dermatomyositis, Diabetes, Drug addiction, Drug Allergies, Dyslexia, Early greying of hair, Eczema, Epilepsy, Gonorrhoea, Hardening of arteries, Hay fever, Heart attack, Hodgkin's disease, Kidney disease, Leukaemia, Liver disease, Migraine, Mental retardation, Multiple sclerosis, Nervous disease or breakdown, Obesity, Operations, Osteoarthritis, Parathyroid disease, Parkinson's disease, Pernicious anaemia, Phobias, Porphyria, Psoriasis, Rheumatoid arthritis, Schizophrenia, Stroke, Suicide, Syphilis, Systemic lupus erythematosis, Thyroid disease, Tuberculosis, Urticaria (hives), Vitiligo.

		YEAR OF BIRTH	AGE AT DEATH	DETAILS
MOTHER				
GRANDMOTHER				
GRANDFATHER				
FATHER				
GRANDMOTHER				
GRANDFATHER				
SISTERS				
BROTHERS				
AUNTS & UNCLES	MOTHER'S SIDE			
	FATHER'S SIDE			

Formatted notepaper

This is simply paper with all the relevant homeopathic headings printed on it. The advantage of using formatted notepaper is that while you remain free to talk about any aspect of the case at any time, the headings will ensure that the basic homeopathic information is always recorded. You are also able to re-format your note paper as your approach to case-taking changes over the years.

The disadvantage of formatted notepaper is that you need to turn the pages to the relevant areas as your patient talks about different aspects of his health. This could be a little off-putting to some patients.

Here is an example of formatted notepaper designed by my student, Dr Dapinder Rattan Singh.

Case Number	
Referred by	
GP	
Date of first consultation	

First Name	
Surname	
Date of Birth	
Age	
Marital Status	

Address

Telephone number

Mobile

Ethnicity/Appearance

Childhood

Family History

Vaccinations/Immunisations

DTP

MMR

Meng C

Flu

Typhoid

Hep A/B

Drug Hx/OTC

PMH/Chronological 'timeline'

Pathology/Investigations

Presenting Complaint/History

Concomitant
Location
Aetiology
Modality
Sensation

Characteristic
SRP

Mental – emotions/understanding/memory

Generals
< > timing
Temperature
Sweat
MODALITIES
Time
Periodicity
Temperature
Weather
Position
Motion
Rest
Touch
Pressure
Sides/Location
Causation/never well since
SENSATIONS
FOOD desire/aversions/thirst

Sexual Function/Desire

Menses

Sleep/Dreams

Particulars

HEAD

EYES

ENT

FACE

MOUTH

GI

GU/GENITALS
URINE

RESP

CVS

MUSCULOSKELETAL

EXAMINATIONS/INVESTIGATIONS

Repertorisation/Rubrics

MIASM: PSORA   TUBERCULOSIS   SYCOSIS   SYPHILIS   CANCER   ACTIVE/EXPOSED/DORMANT

TOTALITY
MIASMATIC
AETIOLOGICAL
SRP
NOSODE
LAYER
PATHOLOGICAL
KEYNOTE

TREATMENT/PRESCRIPTION

1

2

3

100%
90%
80%
70%
60%
50%
40%
30%
20%
10%

MONTHS

Shorthand

A homeopath trained in taking notes in conventional shorthand is able to record the case meticulously as well as maintaining good eye contact with his patient. This is so advantageous that it is quite surprising that shorthand is not taught routinely on all homeopathic training courses.

Homeopathic shorthand

All homeopaths use some form of shorthand. Here are some well-known homeopathic abbreviations:

<	the symptom is aggravated by.
<<	the symptom is strongly aggravated by.
>	the symptom is ameliorated by.
>>	the symptom is strongly ameliorated by
//	the symptom is unaffected by.

Craves sweets + or craves sweets or CRAVES SWEETS.
> You can obviously choose to underline as many times as you want or use any number of plus signs.

I also use the following abbreviations.

MC	the main or presenting complaint
PMH	past medical history
PSH	past surgical history
Vac.	vaccinations
CVS	cardiovascular system
Resp.	lungs and breathing
UGT	urogenital system
GIT	gastrointestinal system
ENT	ear, nose and throat
CNS	central nervous system
GEN	general symptoms
M	mental symptoms
Δ	Medical diagnosis
Med.	current orthodox medications
Hx.	homeopathic prescription
Rx.	orthodox medical prescription

? Puls.   consider Pulsatilla if first choice remedy is inactive
?? Puls.   Pulsatilla may well be needed at some stage in the
           management of this case.

The remedies themselves have conventional abbreviations such as:

Sul.   Sulphur
Nat. mur. Natrum muriaticum

However these may be abbreviated even further, e.g.

NM   Natrum muriaticum

As far as the remedies are concerned, it is fine to abbreviate them in your notes. However many homeopaths consider it poor etiquette to use these abbreviations when discussing a case. It is always better to say 'Magnesium carbonicum' than 'Mag. carb.'. Latin is the official language of homeopathic nomenclature. It is an efficient, elegant and international way of naming our remedies for all homeopaths. If homeopaths of different countries start using their own abbreviated forms of the remedies at international conferences, we will at worst create a homeopathic Tower of Babel and at best eliminate one of the last uses of a fine, classical language.

Computers

I have sat in with a colleague who records all his cases on a computer. As he is able to touch type he can maintain good eye contact with the patient, while occasionally glancing at the monitor. The top half of the screen of the monitor is available for note-taking and the bottom half is used by homeopathic software comprising a sophisticated repertory programme as well as multiple materia medicae which can be 'searched' for any symptom.

There are many other advantages of having all one's cases on a computer. You are able to take all your cases with you whenever you go to a conference or meeting. You can press a button and recall all your cases that have been helped by any remedy you wish to revise or give a lecture on. It becomes a simple matter to e-mail a difficult case (with computer repertory analysis) to colleagues for help. Security and confidentiality are important but are fairly simple to achieve by the use of passwords.

It is important to remember to back up all your cases on a disc or zip drive to avoid a catastrophe, but you can always print out the cases and file them. Some patients may be put off by the technology; expecting a classical homeopath to use a classical pen and paper. However, as the digital generation becomes the majority, there is a good chance that systems like this will become the norm in homeopathy.

Personally, I still enjoy using an old-fashioned fountain pen and unlined, white notepaper. I like the idea of starting each case with a blank sheet of paper. I can draw organs of the body on it to explain things to my patient and add doctors' referral letters and notes from my patient to the file with ease. I always keep drawings made by children with their notes. Of course, I own a computer with all the latest homeopathic software, but I choose to keep it well out of sight of my patients. I also keep my stethoscope, electronic thermometer and blood pressure machine well hidden. I do not find gadgets aesthetically pleasing. They are indispensable but can be kept in desk drawers. For me the ideal setting for the homeopathic conversation is in a room that looks and feels like a comfortable sitting room. The homeopathic books on the shelves have become old friends now and I would miss them if they disappeared into a hard drive. I guess you could say that I am clinging on to the 20th century for a while. I may still become 'digitalised' – but it hasn't happened yet.

Chapter 18

Learning and Teaching Case-taking Skills

Most homeopathic training courses teach their students what sort of information you need to get from taking the history. What is seldom taught is how to get that information.

Students of classical homeopathy all know how important it is to get an accurate, psychological profile of the patient. However this is easier said than done. The art of taking the case in homeopathy is closer to a psychological assessment than it is to the average consultation with a medical doctor. Clinical psychologists will tell you that making such assessments requires a great deal of skill. Acquiring the necessary skills takes training and supervision. A psychotherapy school will routinely include this in its syllabus. Until now homeopathic training courses have not focused on the art of taking the case but there are some encouraging signs that this vital part of the homeopathic process is starting to get more of the attention it deserves. Perhaps this is due to a general swing in homeopathic circles towards the classical approach.

Counselling skills

In Chapter 9 I mentioned how invaluable a short course in Rogerian counselling had been in my education as a doctor and a homeopath. I would advocate the inclusion of similar training programmes in all homeopathic colleges. The course I attended was not aimed specifically at homeopaths and yet I found the theory and especially the practical exercises immensely useful. Teachers of counselling skills could easily be employed to run similar courses as an integral part of all classical homeopathic training programmes. It would not be difficult to explain to these teachers what sort of information we need from our patients. They could then modify their courses in counselling to the requirements of students of classical homeopathy.

Practical exercises

Case-taking is best taught using practical exercises. A simple way of doing this is to divide the class into groups of three. Each trio is given a short exercise to practise a specific exercise in role playing.

An example: The class is told that they are going practise how to deal with a patient who gets very angry while talking about something that happened in the past. Each trio divides itself into three roles: Patient, homeopath and timekeeper/observer. The student designated as 'patient' begins the exercise by role-playing a person who is very angry about a specific issue of their choice. If the 'patient' is prepared to talk about something that really happened to them, the exercise becomes much more powerful. The 'homeopath' listens, reassures or offers tissues; generally doing whatever he thinks would be appropriate in an actual consultation.

When the time allocated for the exercise is over, the timekeeper/observer simply says 'time!'. The 'patient' then spends a couple of minutes giving feedback about how they felt the 'homeopath' handled the situation. Then the 'homeopath' says how he felt the exercise went. Finally the timekeeper/observer gives a more objective opinion of what he saw acted out in front of him. The group then rotates so that each member gets the chance to play each role. The entire exercise can be performed in less than half an hour. A homeopathic tutor can wander among the groups observing the exercise in action. When the exercise has been completed the different groups can share what they have learned with the whole class.

Here are some more examples of exercises to be practised in groups of three students:

- Dealing with a patient with eczema who doesn't understand why he is being asked questions about fears and phobias

- Asking a patient about their libido and sex life

- What to do when a patient breaks down and cries

- Dealing with patients who pester you with regular phone calls, using a couple of mobile telephones as props

- Explaining to the patient how to take the homeopathic medicine prescribed

- A patient returning for the second visit is disappointed at not having improved. He wants to know how many more visits will be required and how much more it is all going to cost him

- A patient is complaining bitterly about an aggravation. The homeopath is not convinced it is a true aggravation at all

- The homeopath feels that the patient needs to see an orthodox doctor for a conventional diagnosis. The patient insists on being treated only with homeopathy

- The homeopath is talking to the mother of a seven-year-old patient with emotional problems. The homeopath suspects that the parents' marriage is on the rocks and this is the reason the child is not getting better

- A patient is clearly attracted to the homeopath and suggests they meet for lunch one day

- The second consultation: role play the scenarios that might be associated with each of the possible reactions to the first prescription. (These are well documented by Kent in his *Lectures on Homoeopathic Philosophy*[80] and by Vithoulkas in *The Science of Homoeopathy.*)[81]

These are all practical examples that occur in the career of every homeopath. Another way of choosing an exercise is for a student to tell the group about a problem he had during a consultation. Each trio then role plays the situation.

Group work

If a homeopathic class comprises 12 students or fewer, it can function as a single group. Larger classes can divide into groups of 8 to 12 students. These groups should meet for at least an hour-and-a-half each month to talk about challenging experiences with patients and share their feelings with the group. The group should ideally be facilitated by a homeopath experienced in working with groups. If such a tutor is not available, the group can still function well with a non-homeopathic facilitator.

Homeopathic training courses may well need to employ a professional group analyst to begin with. As time goes by, the homeopathic tutors (who should be involved in ongoing group work themselves – see the next chapter on supervision) will learn how to facilitate groups themselves. Eventually the course will contain experienced homeopaths trained in working with groups of students.

Video cases

Video cases have been used for many years in homeopathic training but usually to show students' cases that have responded well to a particular remedy. The video camera is inevitably pointed at the patient rather than at the homeopath. Seeing a typical Nux vomica or Platina case is a valuable learning experience. However to learn about taking the case we need to point the camera at the homeopath.

The ideal use of video for this purpose would be to include both patient and homeopath in the picture. Technically it can be tricky to show both faces using a single video camera, but it is the facial expressions and the body language of the homeopath that must take precedence here.

Tutors on video
If the video is of an experienced homeopathic tutor taking a case, it can be highly instructive for that tutor to take the students through the case, explaining his actions and the order of questions. He can stop the video at crucial points of the consultation and ask his students to give their opinions of how he handled that particular moment. The object of the exercise would not be to demonstrate perfection in taking the case. Students should be made to feel free to make constructive criticisms about the way the case was taken. They should also remember that it takes courage for an experienced homeopath to go on video and let everyone see his mistakes.

Student homeopaths on video
Student homeopaths should be required to present at least one video case to their tutors and fellow students. They should be given clear instructions on how to film this particular consultation.

They should be told not to select one of their 'successful cases'. They should rather select a patient, explain to him that the case will be used for teaching purposes and present that particular video whatever the outcome. The case analysis and result of any prescription are not the point here. The whole exercise is about the case-taking itself and for this reason the video camera should be pointed mainly at the student homeopath.

This sort of video exercise is obviously not restricted to the first consultation. It is a good way of teaching students about the follow-up to the first consultation and the second prescription. The ideal video presentation would include the initial consultation and at least one follow-up consultation.

Students could bring videos of their consultations to their class or tutorial group for discussion.

Here are three ways of using these videos to teach case-taking skills.

1. The whole video is shown, but paused at selected times by the tutor. The tutor should feel free to compliment something the student did or said but also to point out 'mistakes' and suggest ways that the situation could have been handled differently. This method has the disadvantage of taking at least an hour. Practically this means that only one video could be used every teaching session.

2. The video is fast-forwarded by the tutor and the class watches randomly selected sections of the case. This method is good for analysing the case but the objective of the exercise is to observe the homeopath rather than the patient. The advantage of this method is that several students' cases can be shown in a single teaching session.

3. Every student is required to hand in a video of himself taking a case to his tutor. The tutor than scans through all the videos in his own time. He is then able to make a selection of segments of consultations he feels will be most useful to teach particular case-taking skills. This is probably the most effective method. Its only disadvantage is that it is extremely time-consuming for homeopathic teachers!

An excellent exercise

Roger Neighbour's *The Inner Consultation*[82] is by far the best book on general practice that I have read. I recommend it as essential reading for all doctors, homeopaths and other health practitioners. He has kindly given me permission to include the following.

In the consultation, there are five places to make for. I call them 'Checkpoints'. They are:

Checkpoint 1: Connecting
Checkpoint 2: Summarising
Checkpoint 3: Handing over
Checkpoint 4: Safety netting
Checkpoint 5: Housekeeping

It's handy that there are five checkpoints, because you need to remember them. Five is literally a 'handy' number, because you've got five digits on a hand. Most children use their fingers when they're learning to count. Many adults, too, tick off their fingers when, for instance, they are making several points in a speech, or trying to recall items from a list they have learned for an exam. For convenience, we'll link the five checkpoints to the fingers and thumb of your left hand as follows

Index finger: Connecting
Middle finger: Summarising
Ring finger: Handing over
Little finger: Safety netting
Thumb: Housekeeping

Memorising exercise
Now is as good a time as any for you to commit these checkpoints to memory. It's important that you involve as many sensory modalities as possible in the act of remembering, so do it this way. First of all look at the figure below:

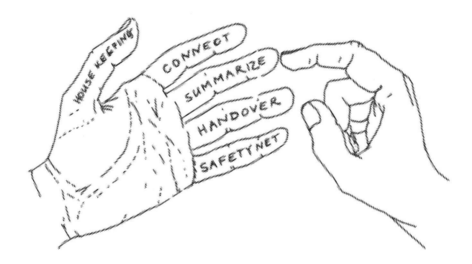

Now place your own left hand in the same position as the one in the figure. In your mind's eye, picture the word 'connect' written on your left index finger. When you can 'see' it, say the word 'connect' out loud a few times and as you do lightly tap the tip of your finger with the index finger of your other hand. In this way you combine the sense modalities of sight, sound and touch with the concept of 'connecting', and imprint them in a single mnemonic, your left index finger.

Use the same 'see, say, tap' sequence to imprint the words:

'Summarise' on to your left index finger
'Hand over' on to the ring finger
'Safety net' on to the little finger
'Housekeeping' on to your thumb

Finally, say the sequence 'Connect, summarise, hand over, safety net, housekeeping' quietly to yourself a few times, looking at each digit in turn as you do, and giving it a tap or two with your right index fingertip. Once or twice in the next half hour, reinforce this learning by ticking off the checkpoints on your let hand's fingers, until you are satisfied that the mnemonic is in place.

And so to summarise: think of the consultation as a journey with five checkpoints to be visited along the way. Taken in order, these checkpoints mark out a route which will accomplish the tasks that are important in the consultation.

I strongly recommend that you take Dr Neighbour's advice and do the exercise he recommends. I did it myself many years ago and the effect has stayed with me ever since.

Now let us explore how these 'checkpoints' can be useful in homeopathic case management.

Checkpoint 1: Connecting
Establish rapport with your patient. There is no one way of doing this as should be clear by now. Every homeopath must embark on a journey to find the way that suits his personality best. Different strategies will be needed in every case. Flexibility of approach is essential.

Checkpoint 2: Summarising

- an empathic talk to the patient about his orthodox, medical diagnosis

- an explanation of how you understand the situation from the homeopathic point of view.

Checkpoint 3: Handing over

- actually giving the patient the homeopathic remedy in the consulting room

- giving the patient a prescription for a homeopathic remedy

- explaining to the patient exactly how and when the remedy should be taken

- answering any questions the patient may have about the homeopathy and homeopathic remedies.

Checkpoint 4: Safety net

- Some homeopaths warn their patients about possible aggravations. I do not do this as it seems to increase the number of 'homeopathic aggravations' experienced by my patients. If a patient asks me specifically about aggravations, I explain that they occur in approximately 10 per cent of cases that eventually do well

- Give the patient your telephone number and ask them to phone you if they have any problem or any question they need answered before the next appointment. This is my chosen form of 'safety netting'. All patients get my mobile-phone number and I have not found myself burdened with too many calls. I realise that a few well-chosen words on the phone can have a therapeutic effect. Occasionally patients phone me at inconvenient hours about mundane matters and in these cases I suggest that my mobile number is really for medical emergencies.

Checkpoint 5: Housekeeping

- regular individual and/or peer group supervision of your cases

- see 'Projective Identification' in Chapter 20, Postgraduate Supervision.

Chapter 19

Talking about Treatment

Although the best consultations feel unrestrained by time, the taking of the case does have to end or at least pause. You may notice that your patient is looking at his watch, perhaps thinking of a parking meter or his next task of the day. A glance at a clock may tell you that the allotted time is coming to an end. It is never a good idea to look at your watch at any stage of the consultation. It may make your patient feel as if he is wasting your time or that you are hinting that he should leave. Hints are inauthentic and should be avoided in homeopathy. Your patient should know in advance approximately how long he is going to spend with you – so there is no reason why you should be embarrassed about telling him that this particular conversation is now at an end.

The case-taking is incomplete

Inevitably, you will occasionally feel that you would like to carry on talking to your patient; that the process of taking the case has not been completed. Hahnemann recognised this natural response when he advocated 'repeated conversations' between homeopath and patient. This is not always due to a lack of time. It may also be due to the patient not yet feeling ready to talk to you about certain areas of his life such as his sex life. At these times, I simply acknowledge what I am feeling and say something like: 'Well, we have had a good chat about your problem but I feel we need to talk some more so that I can get to know you better. I'd like to suggest that you come back soon for another hour. In the meantime, I will think about what you have said.'

As I have mentioned in Chapter 11, some patients will expect treatment after the first consultation and be disappointed if they don't get it. I am sympathetic to such patients but will not allow myself to be pressurised into making an inferior prescription. If I sense that patients feel suspicious of my motives, I simply add the word 'suspicious' (in shorthand) to my notes. It is their symptom, not my problem.

Some homeopaths may choose to prescribe a placebo for such patients. Although I am not against the use of placebos in general, I feel uncomfortable about using one in this particular situation. The patient, although expecting a remedy, is also consciously or unconsciously aware that the consultation is incomplete and that you are unsure of how to treat him. The prescription of a placebo at this point may produce an uncomfortable feeling in both homeopath and patient that will reduce the chances of rapport at the next consultation.

Just as in chess, astute handling of the endgame can make all the difference in homeopathy. The consultation may have apparently 'ended' but case-taking should continue until the patient has left the building. At the very time he thinks that you are not taking the case any more, he may let down his guard and give you the symptom that clinches the diagnosis.

The final question

'Do you have anything you would like to ask me?' is standard for me. What's yours?

Prescribing a remedy

If you feel confident enough to make an immediate prescription, then you should tell your patient that you have decided on the first medicine he needs. It is worth saying 'first' because if this medicine is ineffective the patient will be less inclined to think: 'Now I've tried homeopathy and it hasn't worked either'. It is necessary to explain how he can obtain and how he should take the medicine. This should also be written down because the patient may have been through quite a cathartic process in the consultation and may not be able to remember all the details of how he should take the remedy.

You also need to talk about possible antidotes to the remedy. Whatever your belief in the effect of coffee and menthol (in my experience, it's difficult to antidote the right remedy), you need to talk about these as your patient might have heard or read about them. He will then be surprised if you don't mention them. Time can be saved by having this sort of information printed out and given to the patient at the end of the consultation.

In chronic cases, my preferred method of giving the remedy is to prescribe a series of numbered powders to be taken daily. The first few powders are always placebo. I feel comfortable about using placebo in this way as it can elicit valuable information about the patient. If there is a strong 'aggravation' after the first powder, then you know your patient is very suggestible and you need to be cautious in your interpretation of his response to any subsequent prescription.

Aggravations

I never initiate a conversation about homeopathic aggravations. In the days when I used to do this, many more of my patients suffered from very disturbing 'aggravations' and it was I who was aggravated in the end.

If you mention the possibility of an aggravation, there is a reasonable chance of this acting as a hypnotic suggestion to your patient and he may well feel worse after taking the medicine. It then becomes difficult to differentiate this sort of 'aggravation' from a genuine homeopathic aggravation that confirms the prescription of the right remedy. It is sufficient to tell your patient how to get hold of you if he has any further questions.

If a patient specifically asks you about aggravations or side-effects you are then obliged to say something. I give the following little speech:

'In my experience, about one in ten patients who *do well* on a homeopathic remedy may suffer a mild aggravation after taking the remedy. This is good news as it is usually confirmation that they are taking the right remedy. It seldom lasts for more than two days.'

I say more or less the same thing to patients who are experiencing genuine homeopathic aggravations.

Frequently asked questions about the remedy

These questions seem to come up over and over again. You should have your own answers ready but I've listed the sort of replies I generally use.

Q: What remedy are you giving me?
A: I'll tell you if you really want to know. I would prefer to tell you next time as I don't want you to look it up and think about it. My homeopath never tells me the names of the remedies he gives me until long after I have noticed a good effect.

Q: What does the remedy contain? (Usually asked by patients needing Lachesis or Medorrhinum.)

A: Homeopathic remedies contain extremely small quantities of minerals, metals, plants and even poisons.

Q: Is it safe?

A: Homeopathic medicines are very safe compared to most medicines you could buy over the counter without a doctor's prescription.

Q. How does it act?

A: If the remedy suits you, it can stimulate your body to heal itself. The homeopathic remedy can kick-start that healing ability into action but nobody knows exactly how it manages to do this.

Q: Does it have any side effects?

A: No. However, the right homeopathic remedy works by stimulating your body to heal itself. It cannot tell your body how it should go about fixing itself. Your body heals itself in its own way and the process of healing may leave you with a few unusual sensations. These are not side effects, just what happens to your body as it gets better.

Q: Should I stop taking the doctor's medicine when I start the homeopathic remedy?

A: No. Continue with all your medicines for the time being. Otherwise we won't be able to assess whether the remedy is working. When you improve, we can always wean you slowly off your orthodox medicines. (If you are not the patient's medical doctor, this will need to be done by liaising with the doctor who has prescribed the patient's current medication.)

Q: How long will it take to work?

A: That's hard to say. I've known people to respond in hours and others to take several weeks to improve. If there is no improvement in a month, then we can say that the remedy probably has not acted and we will try to find a better one.

Q: There has been some improvement but how long will it be before I am completely better?

A: It's hard to say. The speed of your improvement is the speed your body is healing itself. The homeopathic remedy just gets the healing process started.

Placebo

This is one of the most controversial subjects in homeopathy. We are interested here only in how the prescription of placebos affects our conversations with patients.

It is terribly difficult for patients to accept that one dose of any medicine can cure them. Those who have studied homeopathy have no problem with a single dose but for most patients this seems ridiculous. Explanations don't really help and if you insist on giving a single dose to most of your patients, you can expect a lot of telephone calls.

Homeopaths have used placebos since the very beginning. Every time a patient takes a placebo he is reminded of the homeopathic consultation and the fact that he is taking a homeopathic remedy. This is therapeutic in itself and a good reason for prescribing a placebo to follow the homeopathic potency.

The problem with prescribing a placebo is that it allows a large element of inauthenticity to enter the homeopath-patient relationship. Every time the patient refers to the placebo as 'the remedy' you may feel a little guilty. We cannot deny that we are being manipulative when we prescribe a placebo. There is also the chance of being 'found out'. This happens more often than you think – and it can be most embarrassing! More than once a patient has asked me directly if I had prescribed a placebo. I was forced to admit it and always felt uncomfortable.

Placebos can be clinically useful for the homeopath and therapeutic for the patient. I sometimes give patients a series of numbered powders with the active remedy in powder 6 or 7, all the rest being placebo. If the patient reacts to powders 1 to 5, I will have learned something about the case. If the reaction comes after the active powder, then I take this as evidence that the remedy is working.

Unfortunately, placebos fail the 'authenticity test' dismally. Occasionally I prescribe the remedy in high potency followed by the same medicine in dosage LM1. This isn't ideal either but at least I don't feel dishonest in the conversations I have with these patients.

What can I say? There seems to be no clear-cut solution to the problem. It is probably best for you to do what feels right for you.

Follow-up consultations

The main subject of these conversations will be the patient's response to the treatment. You need to have a flexible approach to these consultations, as a variety of responses to the remedy is possible. The way a patient may respond to the remedy and what should be done homeopathically has been well described by Kent and graphically illustrated by Vithoulkas. It is worth going through each of these responses and reviewing how you talk to patients in each situation.

It is not only the reaction of the organism to the remedy that is important, but how each individual feels about that reaction. Some patients are immensely grateful for a 20 per cent improvement after a month while others describe a 60 per cent improvement as 'still not completely better'. I always ask patients reporting an improvement to rate it as a percentage.

'If you rate your state of health at zero per cent when you first came to see me and consider 100 per cent as a total elimination of your problem, where would you put yourself now?'

It then becomes possible to plot their improvement on a graph which you can share with them and use to explain each subsequent prescription (see the section on 'formatted notepaper' in Chapter 17)

Unfortunately, as in all branches of medicine, there are those cases that do not respond to the treatment. The conversations we have with these patients are discussed in the final chapter.

Chapter 20

Postgraduate Supervision

All classical homeopaths are students of homeopathy. Different training courses all over the world confer degrees and diplomas on their students but this merely signifies the end of the first stage of study. One's first training course in homeopathy is often fascinating, exhilarating and inspiring. The homeopathic textbooks are full of cases where accurate prescribing led to wonderful cures. Why not expect the same in our own practices?

As you begin to practise classical homeopathy and to take personal responsibility for your patients, it soon becomes clear that homeopathy is not as easy as it appears in the books. Results in the clinic are usually erratic for the beginner. A few failed cases in a row can be quite depressing and can even make us question whether homeopathy really works or whether we are good enough at it to be seeing patients. It becomes painfully obvious that the study of homeopathy is an ongoing process with no end in sight. After a few years in practice, one begins to realise that there is no substitute for the long, learning process of trawling through thousands of clinical cases. One of my first teachers in homeopathy, Dr Marianne Harling, wisely told me that 'it is our patients who teach us homeopathy'. It took the better part of a decade for this advice to sink in, but I eventually got the message.

There will be highs and lows along the way. Just when you thought you were getting nowhere as a practitioner, homeopathy will provide you with an inspiring result to keep you interested. How different this is from conventional medicine. I remember a case I saw as an intern, of a young man who was admitted in a confused and violent state. As he had a high temperature, we decided to do a lumbar puncture which I successfully performed with four white-coated auxiliaries holding the patient down! The results, obtained within the hour, revealed a pneumococcal meningitis. I put up an intravenous line and gave him high doses of penicillin. He eventually made a full recovery from a disease, which is almost always fatal if left untreated. This was a case of a simple diagnosis and treatment leading to a lifesaving intervention. Any doctor seeing the same case would have treated it in the same way or found himself in a lot of trouble if he had not. Sometimes I hanker after the simplicity and elegance of hospital medicine at its best. Sometimes – but not often.

The reason for citing this case is to show that making an orthodox medical diagnosis is often a lot easier than making a homeopathic diagnosis. Most young doctors are capable of diagnosing most of their patients. Specialists in the various disciplines can be consulted for the more complicated cases but these are a small minority. Diagnosis is one thing, effective treatment quite another. An orthodox physician cannot be expected to do anything more for a patient than give the currently accepted treatment for their disease. If it's meningitis, a miracle cure is often at hand. If it's arthritis: 'Well I am sure we can do something to ease the pain at least.' All this makes conventional medicine a lot more simple, if not more satisfying, than classical homeopathy. A doctor can hope to keep up a high standard of making diagnoses and giving the recognised form of treatment for many decades.

In the context of classical homeopathy, diagnosis and treatment are the same thing. If we can find our patient's remedy, we will seldom be disappointed with the result. 'If…' Unfortunately this is easier said than done. There will be many cases where we are unable to find the remedy for a variety of reasons. Unlike the orthodox doctor, we cannot just call on the help of a 'specialist'. We may be able to send some of our failed cases to a more experienced homeopath but mostly we will have to struggle along alone. Or does it have to be alone?

Homeopathic colleges have generally recognised the need for some sort of post-graduate supervision. This may take the form of having an individual supervisor or attending a group 'case conference'. There are two essential components of homeopathic supervision.

• Supervision of the case analysis

• Supervision of the consultation.

Supervision of the case analysis

This is the form homeopathic supervision has traditionally taken. Homeopaths present their difficult or unsolved cases to a more experienced practitioner or to a group of peers, hopefully including some more experienced homeopaths. For practical reasons, the patient is not usually present although this can be very useful if possible. It is also possible to show some of the consultation on video. Each member of the group receives a copy of the case notes or the case is presented using an overhead projector or computer.

The homeopath presenting the case takes his colleagues through his impressions of the case. He might say: 'Fear of high places, underlined three times' which could appear in the notes as '+++'. He will then share with the group his general impression of the patient, his choice of symptoms and his analysis of the case. These days this often includes a computerised repertorisation. He then tells the group what remedy he chose, why he chose it and what ensued. Members of the group are then invited to ask questions and give suggestions of alternative ways of analysing the information presented to prescribe different remedies.

It is possible for a member of the group to come up with an inspired homeopathic diagnosis, which leads to an effective prescription. This can happen when the case has been taken well but the homeopath has failed to find the remedy to suit the information obtained from the patient. However many cases have not responded because the homeopath has not managed to extract the essential homeopathic information from his patient in the process of taking the case. In all these cases supervision of the case analysis will prove to be a fruitless exercise.

Supervision of the consultation

It is possible that the most common reason for an inaccurate prescription is that essential, homeopathic data have not been heard and recorded by the homeopath during the consultation. Supervision of what transpired during the consultation can facilitate a fresh way of viewing the whole case, thereby producing a new set of mentals to be included in the case analysis.

In orthodox general practice, supervision of consultations is a rare phenomenon. The psychoanalyst Michael Balint applied the principles of psychoanalysis to the context of general practice. In 1957 he wrote a book called *The Doctor, His Patient and the Illness* [83] which has become a classic text in the training of general practitioners. It was Balint who first spoke of the importance of anything said by the patient, almost as an afterthought, as they are about to leave the room. For example: 'Oh, by the way, my sex drive has not been up to much lately'. This, as we now know, is likely to be the main reason the patient consulted the doctor.

Balint facilitated groups of general practitioners in which the psychological processes that occurred in the mind of the doctor during the consultation would be discussed openly. As Balint was a Freudian, the concepts of transference and counter-transference are central to the discussion. These 'Balint Groups' have continued to the present day but unfortunately are attended by a small minority of doctors.

The object of this sort of supervision would be to increase rapport between patient and doctor, which always leads to better doctoring in general, if not always to better prescribing. In homeopathy, an improved rapport between homeopath and patient means that the homeopath has a much better chance of acquiring the very sort of information he needs to make an effective prescription. It is therefore reasonable to claim that supervision of the consultation is more necessary in homeopathy than it is in orthodox medicine.

Although conventional doctors do not tend to see the need to have their consultations supervised, the same cannot be said for psychotherapists. Supervision of the psychotherapeutic process has long been a requirement within the profession. Far from being an option, supervision is regarded as a responsibility and a necessary part of continuing professional development to the extent that psychotherapists are unable to get insurance without it. We are finally beginning to realise that this should also be the case in classical homeopathy.

Supervision of the homeopathic consultation is a fairly new concept and I have only had a few years of experience as a supervisee and fewer as a supervisor. What I have seen so far has been inspiring and has led me to believe that psychological supervision of the homeopathic consultation may be the cutting edge that has been missing from most courses in classical homeopathy. It is a subject worthy of more than a single chapter of a book. Still, a book about the homeopathic consultation would be incomplete without a discussion on supervision.

There are a few courses for psychotherapists to train as professional supervisors. At the homeopathic training course I teach on, we now employ a professional trainer of supervisors to work with us as a group of homeopathic tutors. The purpose of this is both to have our own difficult cases supervised and to develop a model of supervision that will be designed specifically for the needs of the classical homeopath. The ideal person to supervise homeopaths would be a professional trained in psychotherapy, the supervision of psychotherapists and classical homeopathy. I have yet to meet such a person but it cannot be long before I do. In the mean time I can say that having my own cases supervised by a psychotherapy supervisor has not only been clinically very useful but even personally liberating and enjoyable.

It was supervision that finally taught me that it is virtually impossible to be 'without prejudice' in how I feel about patients. I have as much chance of achieving this in the consulting room as I do in the world at large. We all have different personalities that are a result both of our inherent constitution and important psychological experiences we have undergone since birth, and perhaps even in utero.

The earlier we have important emotional experiences the more powerful they are in shaping our personalities. We may not be able to articulate powerful emotions when we are babies so these emotions are internalised instead of verbalised and have a long-term effect on the sort of people we become. With unconscious forces like this at play, to be 'without prejudice' becomes an impossible ideal.

If we cannot be without prejudice, then the next best thing we can do is try to become aware of our prejudices ('know yourself') and use them in helping us understand our patients. Psychological supervision of our consultations is an invaluable aid in this journey of understanding.

Counter-transference revisited

In Chapter 7, I mentioned how Dr Charles Kennedy had taught me how to use my own emotions in the consulting room as a diagnostic aid. If I felt anger when talking with a child it was more likely that the child needed Chamomilla than Pulsatilla. Patients needing Lachesis left me feeling overwhelmed and annoyed, Nux vomica patients made me feel a bit aggressive myself and Phosphorus patients brought out strong feelings of warmth and compassion. What I have learned from supervision is that these are all good examples of counter-transference.

On discussing Freud in Chapter 8, we briefly examined the concepts of transference and counter-transference and their relevance to the homeopathic consultation. I would like to look at these terms in more detail as they are vital in the process of supervision.

Charles Rycroft, in *A Critical Dictionary of Psychoanalysis*, defines transference as follows:

1. The process by which a patient displaces on to his analyst feelings, ideas, etc. which derive from previous figures in his life.

2. The state of mind produced by (1) in the patient.

3. Loosely, the patient's emotional attitude towards his analyst. [84]

In a conversation I had with an experienced supervisor of psychotherapists, Tessa Bilder, she was able to embellish this definition. She suggested that the process of transference also includes the patient's beliefs about the analyst and the therapeutic relationship, as well as his attitude and behaviour towards the analyst.

It is important to understand that this process of transference is not peculiar to psychoanalysis and will inevitably take place in all homeopathic consultations. For 'analyst', in the definition above, we can substitute doctor, therapist or homeopath. The difference is that while the process of transference is largely unconscious in general practice and homeopathy, it is an essential part of the therapeutic process in psychoanalysis. By becoming conscious of the process of transference, we can learn a great deal about the psychological state and psychological history of the patient. Obviously this is relevant to the classical homeopath.

Now let us look at Rycroft's definition of counter-transference.

1. The analyst's transference on his patient. In this, the correct sense, counter-transference is a disturbing, distorting element in treatment.

2. By extension, the analyst's emotional attitude towards his patient, including his response to specific items of the patient's behaviour. According to some sources, the analyst can use this latter kind of counter-transference as clinical evidence, ie he can assume that his own emotional response is based on a correct interpretation of the patient's true intentions or meaning. [85]

And that is why I have taken you on a little journey through the land of psychobabble. The classical homeopath too, can indeed 'assume that his own emotional response is based on a correct interpretation of the patient's true intentions or meaning'. It can also help you directly identify the essence of the homeopathic remedy needed by the patient. It is possible that being aware of the process of counter-transference may be just as valuable in classical homeopathy as it is in psychoanalysis. One insightful 'flash' as a result of your awareness of the process of counter-transference, may lead you to think of a remedy for your patient. Of course, you will then have to see if the remedy fits the rest of the case. My experience is that it often does. Your emotional response to your patient is a valuable, diagnostic tool and having your case-taking supervised is one of the ways you can learn to use that tool more effectively.

The process of supervision

Supervision of the homeopathic conversation is a new field in which there are, as yet, no authorities. This is because professional supervisors in psychotherapy are hardly likely to have much knowledge of the mentals of a wide range of homeopathic remedies. Still, my colleagues and I have learned a lot by having some group supervision.

The supervisory sessions – usually a full day – have helped me get to know myself and my patients better. In addition I have looked forward to meeting 'difficult patients' again after gaining some insight into why I regarded them as 'difficult' in the first place. I therefore believe that the ongoing process of supervision is improving my skills as a classical homeopath.

Let us have a look at some of the ways that supervision can be of help to the classical homeopath:

• The homeopath can be made aware of personal material that was stimulated by the consultation with his client.

  If you have a parent who beat you or you experienced cruelty as a child, you may have a strong reaction of fear, anger or disdain towards a patient requiring a remedy like Anacardium. By identifying this type of feeling in yourself (labelling the counter-transference), you may realise that the remedy needed was Anacardium, especially if you remember that you felt the same way with one or two other similar patients who responded well to Anacardium. This not only helps you make diagnoses but also helps you get to know yourself better.

• The homeopath recognises that his patient has cast him in a certain role.

This could be the role of mother-figure or father-figure. Realising this, you may then choose to talk to your patient about his mother or father, thereby creating a good chance of the homeopathic conversation moving up a gear.

- The homeopath feels what his patient is feeling.

  You may have a patient who consistently makes you feel angry even though they are apparently always polite and pleasant during consultations. Supervision of your relationship with this patient may show you that your patient deep down is very angry indeed but not showing it overtly in consultation. They are unconsciously projecting those feelings on to you and leaving you angry instead of themselves. It is useful to know this because you may be able to uncover this suppressed anger in your next consultation with the patient. This conversation may well help you find the patient's remedy. (See the section on Projective Identification later in this chapter.)

- The homeopath has shown that he has been unconsciously defending himself against the transference of the client.

  You may find that you resent seeing a certain patient because you feel drained after they consult you. Tiredness or boredom in the homeopath can also be an indicator that you feel angry inside. Supervision may also show you that your patient is attracted to you or sees you as a mother or father figure. When you understand that you have been unconsciously defending yourself against the unexpressed feelings of your patient, you may feel much less drained by them and more likely to be able to help them homeopathically.

Now you may well be thinking how supervision helps you gain these insights. A supervisor may use a variety of techniques to help you gain insight into your relationships with your patients. Here are some examples that I have either personally experienced or heard of in my conversations with two experienced supervisors. I see no reason why postgraduate homeopaths should not supervise each other using these exercises.

1. The homeopath (supervisee) is asked to sit in the posture of their patient. He is then asked to try to feel what his patient feels. He is then asked simple questions such as: 'What do you need?' or 'What do you think your patient needs?' or 'How does the pain leave you feeling?' You may be surprised by what you reveal about your patient.

2. The homeopath is asked whom his patient reminds him of. This can be very revealing because if the patient reminds you of someone you know

well then your knowledge of that person may help you think of possible remedies for your patient.

3. The homeopath may simply be asked: 'In what ways do you find yourself reacting to your patient?' You may not have thought much about the quality of your relationship with your patient. This simple question can reveal the process of counter-transference, thereby helping you understand what is going on unconsciously in your patient's mind.

4. The supervisor relates his own feelings about the homeopath, his patient or their relationship. He may say things like: 'Why am I feeling sad?' (or angry or bored) or 'Why don't I feel sorry for this (very sick) person?' The supervisor is sometimes able to pick up feelings experienced by the patient *through* the homeopath – without the homeopath experiencing the feeling at all. This sounds a bit fantastic, until you see it happen in front of your eyes and you hear the homeopath confirming the suspicions of the supervisor!

The psychological concept of Projective Identification is useful in understanding these processes and I would like to end this chapter by briefly discussing it and giving an example from a recent day of group supervision facilitated by myself.

Projective Identification

As in projection, the individual deals with emotional conflict or internal or external stressors by falsely attributing to another his or her own unacceptable feelings, impulses or thoughts. Unlike simple projection, the individual does not fully disavow what is projected. Instead the individual remains aware of his or her own affects or impulses but misattributes them as justifiable reactions to the other person. *Not infrequently, the individual induces the very feelings in others that were first mistakenly believed to be there, making it difficult to clarify who did what to whom first.*[86]

The sentence I have put in italics is of special significance in homeopathy. The homeopath may experience strong feelings that he were neither there before the consultation nor expressed verbally by the patient.

A good example of this occurred in a postgraduate homeopathic supervision group I was facilitating very recently.

The homeopathic doctors present had brought some cases (on paper) for supervision but I decided against inviting one of them to present a case. Instead I asked if anyone had recently experienced a moment in the consulting room that had been highly emotionally charged. A doctor immediately recalled such a moment and shared it with the group. Interestingly, she had not thought of bringing this case for homeopathic supervision. However, as she began to describe the case it became clear that the experience (of projective identification) was still very much in her mind.

A teenage boy had been brought in to see her with his mother. He was having tremendous problems at school, had been suspended, had no friends other than some fellow pupils who got a kick out of getting him to throw stones at cars and other delinquent acts. The details of the actual case are not as important here as the emotion that was felt by the homeopathic doctor during the consultation. She used words like 'rage', 'furious' and 'livid' to describe how she was feeling towards her patient. The strong anger she had felt was only too evident to the nine or ten doctors in the supervision group.

I asked her: 'Did you feel like slapping his face?' Nobody in the group could doubt the authenticity in the tone of voice in which she answered 'Yes!'.

'And was he acting in an angry way?' I asked. She replied that he had shown no outward signs of anger at all. He simply sat next to his mother with a body language that indicated boredom, displayed little interest in the proceedings and answered questions monosyllabically or briefly, always with undisguised insouciance and a hint of contempt.

This behaviour, however, was quite sufficient to produce rage in the doctor, which of course had to be totally suppressed during the consultation. So where did her anger come from? She said she had felt no anger at the start of her morning surgery and remembered being in quite a good mood before this particular boy and his mother showed up.

The anger she was feeling clearly belonged to her teenage patient. It had been projected on to her by the passive aggressive behaviour of her patient and she had then identified it as anger towards him.

At this point I asked her if the boy had anything to be angry about. It turned out he had suffered multiple traumas including the death of a sibling. The group quite naturally thought of Staphisagria at this point but

I love to make my students open up their repertories. I suggested that they look up the rubric, 'Anger', in the Mind section of their repertories and glance through the sub-rubrics to see if they could find one that suited what had happened in the consulting room.

Within 30 seconds, a doctor had found an appropriate rubric in the Mind section of her copy of the *Synthesis: Repertorium Homeopathicum Syntheticum 1993*.

Anger – **vex** others; inclined to: **Chin.** kr1 mez. kh,kr1[87]

In the next minute another doctor cited a description of the China teenager from Roger Morrison's *Desktop Guide to Keynotes and Confirmatory Symptoms*:

Touchy, moody, sarcastic idealistic teenagers.[88]

Suddenly China officinalis had emerged as a distinct possibility in the case. We had spent approximately 20 minutes in total on the supervision process. Of course, a prescription of China would be premature at this stage. The doctor would need to talk to the patient again and see if China or Staphisagria or another remedy fitted the case better. It will be interesting to hear what transpires in the case and I will report on this on the website associated with this book. The homeopathic result is paramount but it will also be interesting to hear if the patient's power to annoy his homeopathic doctor will have been diminished by her exploration of the process of projective identification in the supervision group.

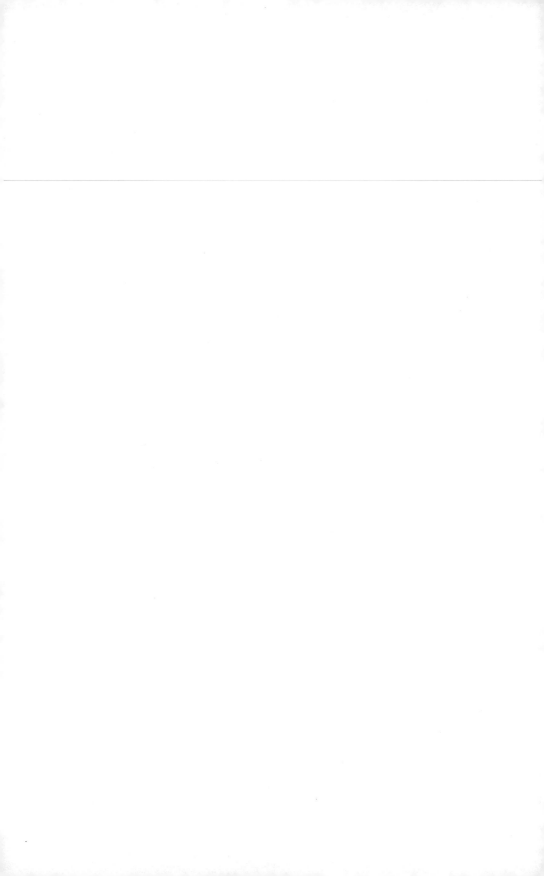

Chapter 21

Saying Good-bye

All conversations have a beginning, a middle and an end and the same is true of the homeopathic conversation. A good consultation can easily be spoiled by a mis-managed conclusion. On the other hand a less productive consultation can often be rescued in the endgame.

It is important to recognise that when you part company with a patient after the first consultation, it is only the end of the first stage of your relationship. You may or may not have prescribed a useful medicine at this point. There is no way of knowing this but it is a good time to remember Hahnemann (it's always a good idea to remember Hahnemann:

> …the physician should endeavour in repeated conversations with the patient to trace the picture of his disease as completely as possible…
> *(Organon §209)*

Your attention has already been drawn to the phrase 'repeated conversations' but I see no harm in repeating it here. Hahnemann knew that we would often need more than one conversation with a patient to get an understanding of him and his disease. The end of the first consultation is an important time but not the moment to judge the success of your relationship with your patient. It is, however, the time to ensure continuity of the homeopathic process.

Keeping in contact

I always give patients a card with my telephone, fax and mobile telephone numbers on it. On the whole, my patients do not misuse this, although one patient faxes me up to ten detailed, typed pages of diary-formatted notes about a week before every appointment. I initially took this as a symptom of Arsenicum album but it was Aurum metallicum that proved to be a useful remedy for him.

I have found the mobile phone very useful. Most of the time it is switched off and acts as a portable answering service. I am then able to hear my patients' messages in their own words. However, I do take calls when I am not consulting as I am aware that patients can be very anxious and a few reassuring words over the phone can be most helpful to them. I don't tend to talk longer than a few minutes as I am not interested in having a consultation on the phone. These tend to be far from satisfactory – homeopathically and financially. However, if a patient moves to another country it is sometimes possible to manage the case on the telephone. This is often the case when you have prescribed a remedy that has acted. I would strongly advise you never to have the first consultation over the phone. As they taught me in medical school – a picture is worth a thousand words.

I don't advise you to encourage patients to e-mail you as this can lead to you receiving regular bulletins on your patients' health. This is not the way to get homeopathic information because it lacks tone of voice, facial expression and appropriate emphasis. I have noticed that there are websites where it's possible to 'consult' a homeopath on the internet. I shudder to think about what Hahnemann would have thought about this. Personally, I would rather have an operation performed on me by a robot, controlled by a surgeon thousands of miles away, than have my case taken via e-mail.

Any fax, e-mail or postcard sent to me by a patient always gets added to the notes. It's all grist to the mill, and it is important to remember to thank a patient for a letter of thanks or a picture postcard.

Failed cases

Every homeopath has cases that do not respond to any of his prescriptions. The conversations we have with patients who keep returning a 'no improvement' verdict on the last prescription can be difficult to handle well. As in all consultations, authenticity is the key. It's best to be totally honest about your thought processes. I often say things like: 'Yes, I agree that your response so far has been disappointing. What I would like to suggest is that I discuss your case with some of my colleagues. Do you mind if I do that? I won't use your real name of course.'

If the patients agree to this (and they all have so far), I take the case to my supervision group.

If a patient says or hints that he is thinking about not coming to see me anymore I might say: 'Yes, I realise that you must be disappointed that you are no better. Still, I feel optimistic that homeopathy will be able to help you.' Or sometimes: 'And you can be sure that if I lose that optimism, if I feel I have run out of good homeopathic ideas, I will tell you I am not interested in banging my head against a brick wall. If it comes to that, I will recommend that you see someone else who can look at your case afresh.'

'Someone else' may be another homeopath or a practitioner of another form of holistic medicine such as acupuncture. It may hurt to give up on homeopathy but the truth is that the patient's remedy may never be discovered in consultation. To a practitioner of traditional Chinese medicine, an examination of the pulses and tongue may yield a clear-cut diagnosis followed by a successful course of treatment. Of course the converse is also true. A patient who does not respond to several treatments of acupuncture may be a clear case of Lycopodium. If only the acupuncturist would send him to a homeopath! We all have to remember that 'the patient comes first' and that means before our own vanity and pride in our work as homeopaths.

'Cured' cases

This is not the place to discuss what is meant by 'cure' but we all see cases where all the original, presenting symptoms are no longer experienced by the patient. When a patient reports this, I ask him to come back immediately if any symptoms recur but in any case to return in six months, even if his illness has not returned. If on this occasion, he is still well, I advise him that an annual chat and check-up could be useful as it allows me to stay in touch with him. If he gets ill, then I don't have to go to the archives to fish out ten-year-old notes.

Strangely enough, only about one per cent of my patients actually take this advice. People don't tend to consult homeopaths when they are feeling well. They may spend a great deal of money on conventional medical checkups and all sorts of orthodox screening tests, but an annual visit to the homeopath who cured them does not seem worthwhile. My teacher, Dr Marianne Harling, gave me the following advice: 'You know that a patient is cured when they have forgotten that it was homeopathy that cured them. And if they forget you, their homeopath, that's a perfect cure.'

I love seeing and chatting to people who have responded well to homeopathy. We all do. Sometimes it's hard to say good-bye, especially to those patients whom you have had the privilege to watch grow stronger as people and start to realise their full potential in life. It is natural to be interested in what happens in their lives when their diseases no longer torment them. We have to accept though that patients do not owe us this, and that we and homeopathy may well be seen as a stepping stone by some patients. Relationships between patients and homeopaths can be very short term, such as in the treatment of an acute illness, or can last a lifetime. It's best not to expect anything and just enjoy one consultation at a time. As William Blake put it in his poem, 'Eternity' [89]

He who binds to himself a joy
Does the winged life destroy:
But he who kisses the joy as it flies
Lives in eternity's sun rise.

Homeopathic consulting, like life itself, has its ups and downs. As we grow more relaxed, tolerant and accepting as people and homeopaths, our consultations tend to become more enjoyable. It's comforting to know that most classical homeopaths continue consulting into their eighties and beyond. This has to be more to do with how much they enjoy their work than the necessity to earn a living!

The time has come for me to say good-bye to you. If you start to enjoy your consultations a fraction more, then this conversation, monologue as it was, will have been worthwhile. My hope is that you and your fellow homeopaths will have many more conversations about the homeopathic conversation.

Appendix

Hippocratic Oath

I swear by Apollo the physician, and Asclepius, and Hygieia (Health) and Panaceia (All-heal) and all the gods and goddesses, making them my witness, that I will fulfil according to my ability and judgment this oath and this covenant:

To hold him who has taught me this art as equal to my parents and to live my life in partnership with him, and if he is in need of money to give him a share of mine, and to regard his offspring as equal to my own brothers in male lineage and to teach them this art – if they desire to learn it – without fee and covenant; to give a share of precepts and oral instruction and all the other learning to my sons and to the sons of him who has instructed me and to pupils who have signed the covenant and have taken an oath according to the medical law, but to no one else.

I will apply dietetic measures for the benefit of the sick according to my ability and judgement; I will keep them from harm and injustice.

I will neither give a deadly drug to anybody if asked for it, nor will I make a suggestion to this effect. Similarly I will not give to a woman an abortive remedy. In purity and holiness I will guard my life and my art.

I will not use the knife, not even on sufferers from stone, but will withdraw in favour of such men as are engaged in this work.

Whatever houses I may visit, I will come for the benefit of the sick, remaining free of all intentional injustice, of all mischief and in particular of sexual relations with both female and male persons, be they free or slaves.

What I may see or hear in the course of the treatment or even outside of the treatment in regard to the life of men, which on no account one must spread abroad, I will keep to myself holding such things shameful to be spoken about.

If I fulfil this oath and do not violate it, may it be granted to me to enjoy life and art, being honoured with fame among all men for all time to come; if I transgress it and swear falsely, may the opposite of all this be my lot.

References

1. Burns, R., *Poems of Robert Burns*, G. Parker (ed.), Midget Classics, n.d.

2. Shem, S., *The House of God*, London: Bodley Head, 1979

3. Leboyer, F., *Birth Without Violence*, London: Fontana/Collins, 1974

4. Gordon-Ross, A.C., *Homeopathy: An Introductory Guide*, Wellingborough: Thorsons Publishers Limited, 1976

5. Hahnemann, S., *Organon der rationellen Heilkunde*, (translated in op. cit., n.20), Dresden: Arnold, 1810

6. Hahnemann, S., *Materia Medica Pura*, R.E. Dudgeon (trans.), London: Hahnemann Publishing Society, 1880

7. Hering, C., *The Guiding Symptoms of our Materia Medica*, Philadelphia: The Estate of Constantine Hering, 1879

8. Allen, T.F., *The Encyclopedia of Pure Materia Medica*, 10 vols, New York, Philadelphia: Boericke & Tafel, 1874–79

9. op. cit., n.7

10. Allen, H.C., *Keynotes and Characteristics with Comparisons*, 2nd edition, Chicago and Philadelphia: Boericke & Tafel, 1899

11. Vithoulkas, G., *Materia Medica Viva*, in progress

12. op. cit., n.6

13. Hughes, R.E.A., *A Cyclopaedia of Drug Pathogenesy*, London: E. Gould and Son, 1886

14. op. cit., n.8

15. Kent, J.T., *Lectures on Materia Medica* (original edition 1904) First Indian edition, Calcutta: M. Bhattacharyya & Co, 1965

16. Kent, J.T., *Lectures on Homoeopathic Philosophy*, Berkeley: North Atlantic Books, 1981

17. op. cit., n.15

18. Kent, J.T., *Repertory of the Homoeopathic Materia Medica*, 5th edition, London: Homoeopathic Publishing Company, 1945

19. op. cit., n.7

20. Hahnemann, S., *Organon of Medicine.* 5th and 6th editions in a single volume (R.E. Dudgeon and W. Boericke, trans. respectively), Philadelphia: Boericke & Tafel, 1922

21. op. cit., n.16

22. Hahnemann, S., *Chronic Diseases Their Specific Nature and Their Homoeopathic Cure*, New York: W.M. Radde, 1845

23. Hahnemann, S., *Lesser Writings*, London: W. Headland, 1851

24. op. cit., n.16

25. Kent, J.T., *What the Doctor Needs to Know In Order To Make a Successful Prescription*, (1900), New Delhi: Jain reprint, 1980

26. Gaier, H., *Thorsons Encyclopaedic Dictionary of Homoeopathy*, London: Thorsons, 1991

27. op. cit., n.22

28. Zaren, A., *Core Elements of the Materia Medica of the Mind*, Volume II, Gottingen: Ulrich Burgdorf Homoeopathic Publishing House, 1993

29. Bailey, P.M., *Homeopathic Psychology*, Berkeley: North Atlantic Books, 1995

30. Coulter, C.R., *Portraits of Homoeopathic Medicines*, Berkeley: North Atlantic Books, 1986

31. op. cit., n.10

32. Clarke, J.H., *A Clinical Repertory to the Dictionary of Materia Medica*, London: Eastern Press Ltd, 1979

33. Clarke, J.H., *A Dictionary of Practical Materia Medica*, London: Homoeopathic Publishing Company, 1901

34. Ledermann, E.K., *Philosophy and Medicine*, 2nd edition, Aldershot: Gower, 1986

35. Ledermann, E.K., *Existential Neurosis*, London: Butterworth & Co, 1972

36. Ledermann, E.K., *Medicine For The Whole Person*, Shaftesbury: Element Books, 1997

37. Rowan, J., *The Transpersonal*, London: Routledge, 1993

38. op. cit., n.16

39. op. cit., n.15

40. op. cit., n.18

41. op. cit., n.16

42. Winston, J., *The Faces of Homœopathy*, Wellington: Great Auk Publishing, 1999

43. Brown, A., *Are You Looking at Me, Jimmy?* Wallington: Methuen 1994

44. Freud, S., *The Interpretation of Dreams*, Volume 4, Harmondsworth: Pelican, 1976

45. Ball, P., *10,000 Dreams Interpreted*, Kettering: BK Index,1996

46. Shakespeare, W., *Complete Works*, Oxford: Oxford University Press, 1974

47. De Witt, C. and J. Baldwin, 'Some Philosophical and Psychological Contributions to the Use of Self in Therapy', *in The Use of Self in Therapy*, M. Baldwin and V. Satir (eds), New York: The Haworth Press, 1987

48. Hawkins, P. and R. Shohet, *Supervision in the Helping Professions*, Buckingham: Open University Press, 1999

49. Whitmont, E.C., *Psyche and Substance. Essays on Homeopathy in the Light of Jungian Philosophy*, Richmond: North Atlantic Books, 1980

50. Stone, H., *Embracing Your Inner Critic*, Harper Collins, 1993

51. Buber, M., *I and Thou*, R.G. Smith (trans.), Edinburgh: T. & T. Clark, 1937

52. op. cit., n.47

53. Rogers, C.R., *The Clinical Treatment of the Problem Child*, Boston: Houghton Mifflin, 1939

54. Rogers, C.R., *Counseling and Psychotherapy*, Boston: Houghton, 1942

55. Baldwin, M., 'Interview With Carl Rogers on the Use of Self in Therapy', in Baldwin and Satir, *The Use of Self in Therapy*, op. cit., p49

56. ibid., p46

57. op. cit., n.18

58. op. cit., n.15

59. Rogers, C.R., *On Encounter Groups*, Harmondsworth: Penguin 1973

60. op. cit., n.46

61. Farrelly, F. and J. Brandsma, *Provocative Therapy*, Cupertino: Meta Publications, 1974

62. Blake, W., *Selected Poetry*, W.H. Stevenson (ed.), London: Penguin Books, 1954

63. op. cit., n.33

64. Clarke, J.H., *The Prescriber: a dictionary of the new therapeutics*,
London: Keene & Askwell, 1885

65. Houghton-Hawksley, H.S. and A.B.S. Eaton (eds), *Wild Wave*,
London: John Murray, 1986

66. Krishnamurti, J., *The First and Last Freedom*, London, 1954

67. Herscu, P., *The Homeopathic Treatment of Children: Pediatriac Constitutional Types*,
Berkeley: North Atlantic Books, 1991

68. op. cit., n.3

69. Wynne-Simmons, A., *The Children's Toy Box: A Search for the Constitutional Remedy in Children*,
London: British Homoeopathic Association, 1993

70. Grandgeorge, D., *The Spirit of Homeopathic Medicines: Essential Insights to 300 remedies*,
Berkeley: North Atlantic Books, 1998

71. op. cit., n.42

72. Rycroft, C., *A Critical Dictionary of Psychoanalysis*, London: Penguin, 1995

73. Campbell, A., *The Two Faces of Homoeopathy*, London: Robert Hale Ltd, 1984

74. op. cit., n.15

75. Hughes, R.E.A., *A Cyclopaedia of Drug Pathogenesy*, London: E. Gould and Son, 1886

76. Boericke, W., *Pocket Manual of Homeopathic Materia Medica and Repertory*,
9th edition, New York: Boericke & Runyon, 1927

77. Harling, M., 'Homoeopathy a la mode', *Homeopathy*, Jan/Feb 1980

78. Sohn, F.W.P.H., *Musik in der Homoopathie*, New York: Barthel & Barthel, 1996

79. op. cit., n.22

80. op. cit., n.16

81. Vithoulkas, G., *The Science of Homoeopathy*, New York: Grove Press Inc, 1980

82. Neighbour, R., *The Inner Consultation*,
Lancaster: MTP Press, 1989 Reprinted by the Petrroc Press, UK, 1997

83. Balint, M., *The Doctor, His Patient and The Illness*,
London: Pitman Medical Publishing, 1957

84. op. cit., n.72

85. ibid.

86. American Psychiatric Association, *Diagnostic and Statistical Manual of Mental Disorders IV*,
Washington DC, 1994

87. Schroyens, F. (ed.), *Synthesis: Repertorium Homeopathicum Syntheticum*,
Brussels: Homeopathic Book Publishers and Archibel SA, 1993, p9

88. Morrison, R., *Desktop Guide to Keynotes and Confirmatory Symptoms*,
Albany: Hahnemann Clinic Publishing, 1993

89. op. cit., n.62

Bibliography

Allen, H.C., *Keynotes and Characteristics with Comparisons*,
2nd edition, Chicago and Philadelphia: Boericke & Tafel, 1899

Allen, T.F., *The Encyclopedia of Pure Materia Medica*, 10 vols, New York, Philadelphia: Boericke & Tafel, 1874–79

American Psychiatric Association, *Diagnostic and Statistical Manual of Mental Disorders IV*, Washington DC, 1994

Bailey, P.M., *Homeopathic Psychology*, Berkeley: North Atlantic Books, 1995

Baldwin, M., 'Interview With Carl Rogers on the Use of Self in Therapy', *in The Use of Self in Therapy*,
M. Baldwin and V. Satir (eds), Haworth Press: New York, 1987

Balint, M., *The Doctor, His Patient and the Illness*, London: Pitman Medical Publishing, 1957

Ball, P., *10,000 Dreams Interpreted*, Kettering: BK Index, 1996

Blackie, M., *Classical Homoeopathy*, E.C.E.A.F. Johnson (ed.), Beaconsfield: Beaconsfield Publishers Ltd, 1986

Blake, W., *Selected Poetry*, W.H. Stevenson (ed.), London: Penguin Books, 1954

Bodman, F., *Insights into Homoeopathy*,
A. Davies and R. Pinsent (eds), Beaconsfield: Beaconsfield Publishers Ltd, 1990

Boericke, W., *Pocket Manual of Homeopathic Materia Medica and Repertory*,
9th edition, New York: Boericke & Runyon, 1927

Brown, A., *Are You Looking at Me, Jimmy?* Wallington: Methuen, 1994

Buber, M., *I and Thou*, R.G. Smith (trans.), Edinburgh: T. & T. Clark, 1937

Burns, R., *Poems of Robert Burns*, G. Parker (ed.), Midget Classics, n.d.

Calnan, J., *Talking with Patients – a Guide to Good Practice*, London: William Heinemann Medical Books, 1983

Campbell, A., *The Two Faces of Homoeopathy*, London: Robert Hale Ltd, 1984

Clarke, J.H., *A Dictionary of Practical Materia Medica*, London: Homoeopathic Publishing Company, 1901

Clarke, J.H., *A Clinical Repertory to the Dictionary of Materia Medica*, London: Eastern Press Ltd, 1979

Clarke, J.H., *The Prescriber: a dictionary of the new therapeutics*, London: Keene & Askwell, 1885

Coulter, C.R., *Portraits of Homoeopathic Medicines*, Berkeley: North Atlantic Books, 1986

De Witt, C. and J. Baldwin, 'Some Philosophical and Psychological Contributions to the Use of Self in
Therapy', *in The Use of Self in Therapy*, M. Baldwin and V. Satir (eds), The Haworth Press: New York, 1987

Detinis, L., *Mental Symptoms in Homoeopathy*, Beaconsfield: Beaconsfield Publishers Ltd, 1990

Farrelly, F. and J. Brandsma, *Provocative Therapy*, Capitola: Meta Publications, 1974

Foubister, D., *Tutorials on Homoeopathy*, Beaconsfield: Beaconsfield Publishers, 1989

Freud, S., *Introductory Lectures on Psychoanalysis*. Volume 1, Harmondsworth: Pelican, 1975

Freud, S., *The Interpretation of Dreams*. Volume 4, Harmondsworth: Pelican, 1976

Gaier, H., *Thorsons Encyclopaedic Dictionary of Homoeopathy*, London: Thorsons, 1991

Gemmel, D., *Everyday Homoeopathy*, Beaconsfield: Beaconsfield Publishers Ltd, 1987

Gibson, D.M., *Studies of Homoeopathic Remedies*, Beaconsfield: Beaconsfield Publishers Ltd, 1987

Gordon-Ross, A.C., *Homoeopathy. An Introductory Guide*, Wellingborough: Thorsons Publishers Limited, 1976

Grandgeorge, D., *The Spirit of Homeopathic Medicines: Essential Insights to 300 Remedies,*
Berkeley: North Atlantic Books, 1998

Haehl, R., *Samuel Hahnemann: His Life and Work,* Delhi: B.Jain, 1995

Hahnemann, S., *Chronic Diseases: Their Specific Nature and Their Homoeopathic Cure,*
New York: W.M. Radde, 1845

Hahnemann, S., *Lesser Writings,* London: W. Headland, 1851

Hahnemann, S., *Materia Medica Pura,* R.E. Dudgeon (trans.), London: Hahnemann Publishing Society, 1880

Hahnemann, S., *Organon of Medicine.* 5th and 6th editions in a single volume
(R.E. Dudgeon and W. Boericke, trans. respectively), Philadelphia: Boericke & Tafel, 1922

Harling, M., 'Homoeopathy a la mode', *Homoeopathy,* Jan/Feb 1980

Hawkins, P. and R. Shohet, *Supervision in the Helping Professions.* 1999, Buckingham: Open University Press, 1999

Hering, C., *The Guiding Symptoms of our Materia Medica,*
Philadelphia: The Estate of Constantine Hering, 1879

Herscu, P., *The Homeopathic Treatment of Children: Pediatric Constitutional Types,*
Berkeley: North Atlantic Books, 1991

Hippocrates, *Hippocratic Writings,* Harmondsworth: Penguin, 1987

Houghton-Hawksley, H.S. and A.B.S. Eaton (eds), *Wild Wave,* John Murray: London, 1986

Hughes, R.E.A., *A Cyclopaedia of Drug Pathogenesy,* London: E. Gould and Son, 1886

Kent, J.T., *What the Doctor Needs to Know in Order to Make a Successful Prescription (1900),* New Delhi: Jain, 1980

Kent, J.T., *Repertory of the Homoeopathic Materia Medica,*
5th edition, London: Homoeopathic Publishing Company, 1945

Kent, J.T., *Lectures on Materia Medica (1904),* Calcutta: M. Bhattacharyya & Co, 1965

Kent, J.T., *Lectures on Homoeopathic Philosophy.* Berkeley: North Atlantic Books, 1981

Krishnamurti, J., *The First and Last Freedom,* London, 1954

Leboyer, F., *Birth Without Violence,* London: Fontana/Collins, 1974

Ledermann, E.K., *Existential Neurosis,* London: Butterworth & Co, 1972

Ledermann, E.K., *Mental Health and Human Conscience: The True and False Self,* Amersham: Avebury, 1984

Ledermann, E.K., *Philosophy and Medicine,* 2nd edition, Aldershot: Gower, 1986

Ledermann, E.K., *Medicine For The Whole Person,* Shaftesbury: Element Books, 1997

Ledermann, E.K., *Medicine for the Whole Person. A Critique of Scientific Medicine.*
Rockport: Element Books, 1987

Lloyd, G.E.R. (ed.), *Hippocratic Writings,* Penguin: Harmondsworth, 1950

Lockie, A., *The Family Guide to Homeopathy: The Safe Form of Medicine for the Future,*
2nd edition, London: Hamish Hamilton, 1988

Lockie, A., *Encyclopodia of Homeopathy,* London: Dorling Kindersley, 2000

Martin, P., *The Sickening Mind,* London: Flamingo, 1998

Meares, M., *A Way of Doctoring,* Melbourne, 1985

Mendelf, D., *Proper Doctoring,* Berlin: Springer-Verlag, 1984

Morrison, R., *Desktop Guide to Keynotes and Confirmatory Symptoms,* Albany: Hahnemann Clinic Publishing, 1993

Neighbour, R., *The Inner Consultation.* 1989, Lancaster: MTP Press, 1989, and Petroc Press UK, 1997

O'Connor, J. and J. Seymour, *Introducing Neuro-Linguistic Programming,* Bodmin: Hartnolls Ltd, 1990

Rogers, C.R., *The Clinical Treatment of the Problem Child,* Boston: Houghton Mifflin, 1939

Rogers, C.R., *Counseling and Psychotherapy,* Boston: Houghton, 1942

Rogers, C.R., *On Encounter Groups*, Harmondsworth: Penguin, 1973

Rowan, J., *The Transpersonal*, London: Routledge, 1993

Rycroft, C., *A Critical Dictionary of Psychoanalysis*, London: Penguin, 1995

Sanders, K., *Nine Lives. The Emotional Experiences in General Practice*,
Oxford: The Roland Harris Educational Trust, 1991

Schroyens, F. (ed.), *Synthesis: Repertorium Homeopathicum Syntheticum 1993*,
Homeopathic Book Publishers and Archibel S.A.: Brussels, 1993

Shakespeare, W., *Complete Works*, Oxford: Oxford University Press, 1974

Shem, S., *The House of God*, London: Bodley Head, 1979

Singer, C., *A Short History of Medicine*, Oxford: Oxford University Press, 1928

Sohn, F.W.P.H., *Musik in der Homoopathie*, New York: Barthel & Barthel, 1996

Stone, H. and S. Winkleman, *Embracing Ourselves*, Marina del Rey: Devorrs & Co, 1985

Stone, H., *Embracing Your Inner Critic*, London: Harper Collins, 1993

Thorne, B., *Carl Rogers*, London: Sage, 1992

Vithoulkas, G., *The Science of Homoeopathy*, New York: Grove Press Inc, 1980

Whitmont, E.C., *Psyche and Substance. Essays on Homeopathy in the Light of Jungian Philosophy*,
Richmond: North Atlantic Books, 1980

Winston, J., *The Faces of Homœopathy*, Wellington: Great Auk Publishing, 1999

Wynne-Simmons, A., *The Children's Toy Box: A Search for the Constitutional Remedy in Children*,
London: British Homoeopathic Association, 1993

Zaren, A., *Core Elements of the Materia Medica of the Mind*,
Volume II, Gottingen: Ulrich Burgdorf Homeopathic Publishing House, 1993

NOTES